Essential surgical

technique

Essential surgical technique

Edited by

Colin D. Johnson MChir, FRCSEng

University Surgical Unit, Southampton General Hospital,
Southampton, UK

and

John Cumming ChM, FRCSEdin

Department of Urology, Southampton General Hospital,
Southampton, UK

CHAPMAN & HALL MEDICAL

London · Weinheim · New York · Tokyo · Melbourne · Madras

Published by Chapman & Hall, 2-6 Boundary Row, London SE1 8HN, UK

Chapman & Hall, 2-6 Boundary Row, London SE1 8HN, UK

Chapman & Hall GmbH, Pappelallee 3, 69469 Weinheim, Germany

Chapman & Hall USA, 115 Fifth Avenue, New York, NY 10003, USA

Chapman & Hall Japan, ITP-Japan, Kyowa Building, 3F, 2-2-1 Hirakawacho, Chiyoda-ku, Tokyo 102, Japan

Chapman & Hall Australia, 102 Dodds Street, South Melbourne, Victoria 3205, Australia

Chapman & Hall India, R. Seshadri, 32 Second Main Road, CIT East, Madras 600 035, India

First edition 1997

© 1997 Chapman & Hall

Typeset in Best-set Typesetter Ltd., Hong Kong
Printed in Great Britain at The Alden Press, Osney Mead, Oxford

ISBN 0 412 55470 4

A Catalogue record for this book is available from the British Library

Library of Congress Cataloging-in-Publication Data available

∞ Printed on acid-free text paper, manufactured in accordance with ANSI/NISD 239.48–1992 (Permanence of Paper)

Contents

Contributors

Louise E. Allen FRCOphth
Department of Ophthalmology, Addenbrookes NHS Trust,
Cambridge, UK

Hugh J. Clarke FRCSEng
Department of Orthopaedic Surgery, Queen Alexandra Hospital,
Portsmouth, UK

John Cumming ChM FRCSEdin
Department of Urology, Southampton General Hospital,
Southampton, UK

Mervyn Griffiths MCh FRCSEng
Wessex Regional Centre for Paediatric Surgery, Southampton
General Hospital, Southampton, UK

Colin D. Johnson MChir FRCSEng
University Surgical Unit, Southampton General Hospital,
Southampton, UK

Mohammed A. Khan FFAEM
Accident and Emergency Unit, Southampton General Hospital,
Southampton, UK

J. Knighton
Department of Anesthesiology, University of Michigan Hospital,
Michigan, USA

Dorothy A. Lang FRCSEng
Wessex Neurological Centre, Southampton General Hospital,
Southampton, UK

Brian A. Leatherdale BSc, MD, FRCPLond
Royal South Hants Hospital, Southampton, UK

Peter D. Lees MS, FRCSEng
Wessex Neurological Centre, Southampton General Hospital,
Southampton, UK

Christopher J. Randall FRCSEng
Department of ENT, Southampton General Hospital, Southampton, UK

Andrew J. T. Sansome FCAnaes
Department of Anaesthesia, Southampton General Hospital, Southampton, UK

Rodger A. Sleet FRCPEdin FRCGP FFAEM
Accident and Emergency Unit, Southampton General Hospital, Southampton, UK

Victor T. Tsang MS, MSc, FRCSEng
Wessex Cardiothoracic Unit, Southampton General Hospital, Southampton, UK

David Weeden FRCSEng
Wessex Cardiothoracic Unit, Southampton General Hospital, Southampton, UK

Andrew D. Wilmshurst FRCSEng
Department of Plastic Surgery, Dundee Royal Infirmary, Dundee, UK

Preface

This book addresses the needs of the newly defined basic surgical trainee. Most BSTs now take part in prolonged rotations, with relatively brief exposure to a wide range of different specialties. This book is designed to go with the trainee through the rotation, to provide a practical guide to the procedures that s/he may be expected to perform in each specialty.

The Editors have deliberately avoided including major procedures at which the BST will be an interested observer. The emphasis throughout is on a clear practical guide to the minor and intermediate procedures which the trainee will perform. Undoubtedly, the first attempts at most of these procedures will be well supervised, but we hope that the descriptions in this book will help the trainee to master each procedure rapidly and with confidence.

In addition we have included chapters on general aspects such as medical management, local anaesthetic techniques and basic surgical skills such as knot tying and instrument handling.

We have adopted a direct, didactic style, because basic surgical trainees need clear direction. There are of course many other ways of doing most of the procedures described in these pages, and such variations will doubtless stimulate helpful discussions on practical points. Discussion and justification have been kept to a minimum, because we have focused on the essential practical steps of the procedures described.

We feel this book will meet a need felt by basic surgical trainees, who look for clear guidance in practical aspects of a variety of clinical disciplines.

C. D. Johnson
J. Cumming
Southampton, 1997

Surgical skills

1

Colin D. Johnson

The feature that sets apart surgeons from other doctors is the ability to operate on or inside the body of the patient, to remove diseased tissues or to rearrange the internal anatomy. These manipulations require a variety of surgical skills, the most basic of which are common to all surgical specialties. In the chapters that follow you will read how to perform a large number of surgical operations. This chapter concentrates on the various skills you will have to put together in order to carry out these procedures.

SUTURE MATERIAL

The first time you go to the operating theatre as a surgeon rather than as an interested onlooker, you will have to answer the nurse's question: what suture would you like? It is as well to think about this beforehand in order to avoid an embarrassing silence or a hasty choice of the wrong material. Under some circumstances your consultant will have laid down a clearly defined policy. Follow such policies.

Sutures are of two main types of material, absorbable or non-absorbable, and of two main types of manufacture, braided and monofilament. In general, natural and braided absorbable sutures are absorbed more rapidly than synthetic monofilament sutures. Natural braided non-absorbable sutures are more prone to harbour infection than synthetic monofilament non-absorbable sutures. Some of the types available are shown in Table 1.1.

Braided suture materials are easier to handle and to tie. They are often used for situations where precision is important, as in skin suture and intestinal anastomosis. Non-absorbable sutures are used internally when continuing long-term strength is important, for example in hernia repair. Many surgeons prefer monofilament material for the skin because it is less prone to cause infection. Chromic catgut is now obsolete. You should only use it if your consultant expressly instructs you to do so. It has a short time to absorption, so it loses strength rapidly in the tissues; it can cause an inflammatory reaction, as it is foreign protein; and it should only be used where this

Table 1.1   Types of suture

	Braided	*Monofilament*	*Absorbable*
Natural			
Linen	✓		No
Silk	✓		No
Catgut		✓	Yes
Synthetic			
Vicryl	✓		Yes
Dexon	✓		Yes
PDS		✓	Yes
Nylon	✓	✓	No
Polypropylene		✓	No

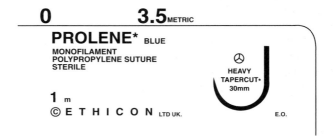

Fig. 1.1   A typical suture pack. This clearly indicates the needle shape and size. The style of tip is printed beneath the needle. The suture material is colour-coded and printed on the pack. Suture thickness is indicated in two styles (metric numbers increase with increasing thickness whereas increasing numbers in the style 00, 000 or 2/0,3/0 indicate progressively finer sutures). There is also a specific manufacturer's code that signifies the exact type of needle and suture.

effect is unlikely to cause harm and where rapid dissolution is an advantage.

Suture packs

It is helpful to understand the information printed on the outside of the suture pack. A commonly used format is explained in Fig. 1.1.

From the pack you can identify the type of needle and its size, the length and thickness of the suture material and any other special features. If two needles are shown the suture is 'double-ended', i.e. it has a needle swaged on both ends. Some sutures are packed two to a pack, and ties are packed in bundles of 10 or 12. The presence of buttress tubes, or buttons or beads to secure the suture, is also clearly marked on the pack.

In many theatres, sutures are referred to by the manufacturer's code number. While this is a convenient shorthand, it can lead to confusion if the code is remembered wrongly. Get into the habit of asking for sutures by their specific description: 'a 2/0 Vicryl suture on a 30 mm round-bodied needle, please'.

SURGICAL KNOTS

The first surgical skill acquired by virtually every medical student and house officer is how to tie a surgical knot. There are numerous variations of this technique, which rely on the principle of wrapping one end of a thread around another thread while holding the 'long' end in one hand and tying the knot with the other hand using the 'short' end. The commonest knot is the triple single throw, which is equivalent to one and a half reef knots. Two ways of applying a single throw are shown in Fig. 1.2. Take care when tightening the knot to maintain tension in the correct direction and evenly between your two hands, so that the knot is tied 'square'.

The surgeon's knot

This knot is tied with a double throw on the first throw, and is completed with two single throws. The double throw helps to prevent the first throw from slackening while the second throw is made (Fig. 1.3).

An even more secure knot is a triple double throw, which is quite adequate for any synthetic monofilament material. The technique of this is shown in Fig. 1.3.

Slip knot

When there is some elasticity in the tissues, leading to slackening of the first throw of the knot, it is useful to tie a slip knot. This knot is particularly useful for suturing the skin with interrupted monofilament sutures. Tie a single throw of the knot but do not tighten it fully. Maintain tension on the long thread and tie another throw around this in the opposite direction to the first throw. By maintaining tension on the 'long end' thread you will produce a double half-hitch, which can then be slid down to the required tension (Fig. 1.4). This should then be followed by two 'square' throws, in order to prevent the slip knot from slipping undone.

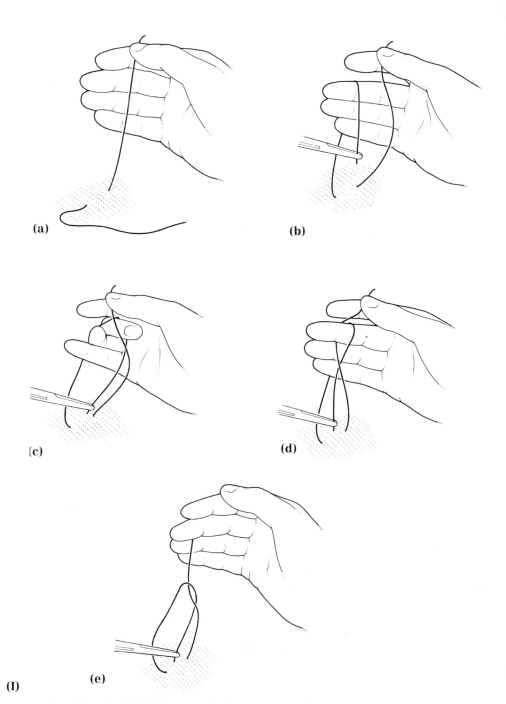

(a)

(b)

(c)

(d)

(e)

(I)

Fig. 1.2 **(I) (a)** Hold one end of the suture fixed in one hand. **(b)** Hold the loose end between the finger and thumb of your dominant hand, with the palm facing towards you and the end of the thread over the thenar aspect of the index finger. Extend the middle and ring fingers and lay the thread over them. **(c)** Next, take the fixed thread around the dorsal aspect of the middle and ring fingers and bring it back over the palmar aspect of these fingers at

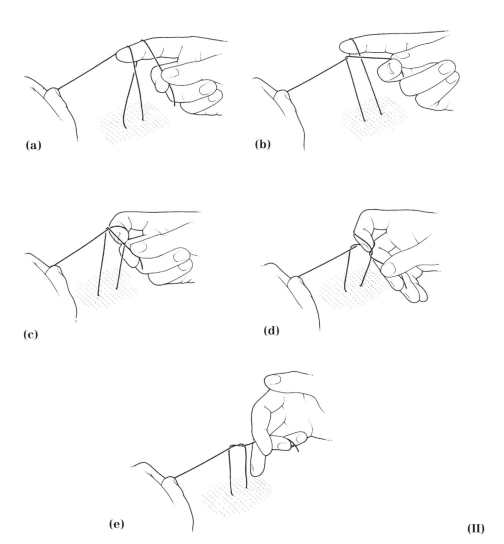

(a)

(b)

(c)

(d)

(e)

(II)

the level of the distal interphalangeal joint. **(d)** Flex the middle finger and hook it inside the loose thread, held taut by the thumb and index finger. You may find it helpful to use your little finger as well, to hold the thread away from the other two fingers. **(e)** Straighten your middle finger in front of the loose thread so that it passes between the middle and ring fingers. Grasp the thread between these two fingers and let go with your finger and thumb. Slide the fingers out the loop and you will have a single throw. **(II)** Follow on immediately into the second throw. **(a)** Grasp the loose end with the finger and thumb of your dominant hand and extend the middle finger next to the index. **(b)** Adjust your grip to hold the thread between thumb and middle finger and separate the index finger to apply tension to the thread. **(c)** This should run from your grip with thumb and middle finger over the palmar aspect of the index finger and down behind it. **(d)** Lay the fixed end of thread over the pulp of the index finger and then flex this finger to get behind the loose thread. **(e)** As you flick this loop through by extending your index finger let go of the free end and pull it through to form the second throw. This final movement is easier if you grasp the free end of the thread between index and middle fingers.

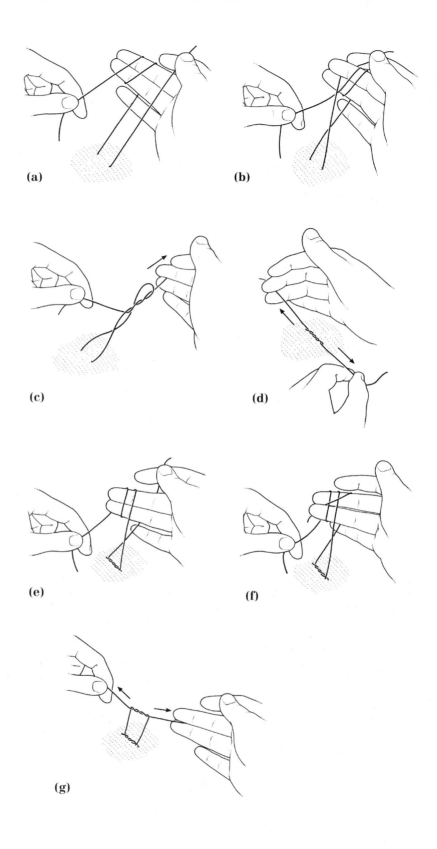

(a)

(b)

(c)

(d)

(e)

(f)

(g)

Tying with instruments

The same knots can be tied using instruments rather than your fingers. The technique is rather different, in that the 'long end' thread is wrapped around the 'short end' thread, rather than the other way round. This is achieved by wrapping the thread around an instrument first, then grasping the 'short end' thread in the instrument and sliding the throws of the knot off the instrument on to the thread. The knot is then tightened (Fig. 1.5). This technique can be applied in any number of combinations to produce the knots described above.

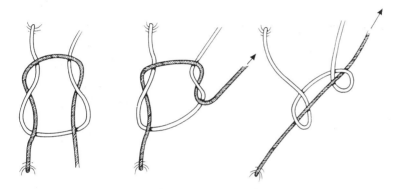

Fig. 1.4 Slip knot. The action is identical for two opposite single throws, but tension (arrow) on the fixed end of the thread produces a slip knot, which can be set to the desired tension.

Fig. 1.3 **(a)** After tying the first throw in the usual way with the right hand, hold open the loop with the middle finger of the left hand. **(b)** Pass the middle finger of the right hand back into the loop to pick up the loose end and draw it through again. **(c)** Hold the loose end between your index finger and thumb and pass it across the volar aspect of your middle and ring fingers. Wrap the long ends twice around these fingers in a clockwise direction. **(d)** Curl up the middle finger to catch the loose end and draw it through the loop. **(e)** After tightening the loop as shown in **(c)** and **(d)**, hold the loose end between your index finger and the thumb again but this time pass the loop behind your middle and ring fingers. Encircle these two fingers twice in a counterclockwise direction holding the long end in your left hand. **(f)** Pass the short end down between your middle and ring fingers, grasp the end and **(g)** pull it through the loops. You can also tie a third double throw as shown in **(c)** and **(d)**.

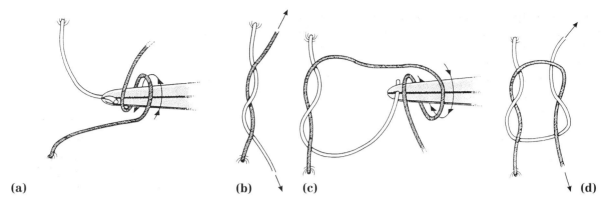

(a)   **(b)**   **(c)**   **(d)**

Fig. 1.5 Instrument ties. Wrap the long end of thread around the tips of a needle holder or artery clip. Grasp the short end in the tips of the instrument **(a)**. Slide the loops off the clip and tighten the knot **(b)**. Then repeat this in the opposite direction to complete a square knot **(c)** and **(d)**.

Specialized knots

The techniques described above will enable you to tie a satisfactory range of basic surgical knots. In different specialties you will be shown how to tie particular knots for special circumstances. It is beyond the scope of this chapter to describe these knots in detail.

SURGICAL INSTRUMENTS

While it may seem obvious how to use surgical instruments, there are particular techniques that can help to improve your use of them. Confident use of the knife will produce a clean wound and will allow rapid progress. Scissors should be used for cutting and not for stretching and tearing tissue. Correctly applied clips or artery forceps will make haemostasis easy and secure and specialized clips can help in dissection and isolation of neurovascular structures. Surgical forceps allow the extension of your fingers into the operating field in a way that produces tactile sensitivity and secure handling of tissue.

Knife

The surgical scalpel comes in one of two forms (Fig. 1.6).

The straight-pointed blade is used only to make small incisions for limited access. This is needed for procedures such as avulsion of varicose veins, insertion of laparoscopic cannulas or placement of chest drains. The curved blade is used in most circumstances, and is designed to allow smooth incision of the tissues.

Hold the scalpel handle in the palm of your hand and rest your index finger along the back of the handle towards the blade. Apply gentle pressure, sufficient to push the blade into the skin, then draw the scalpel smoothly in a straight line for the desired distance. Aim to maintain the lowest point of the blade just below the deep layers of the skin; this will produce a clean cut of consistent depth (Fig. 1.6). Try to achieve this same action of consistent depth and even pressure in all layers of the incision. Incise the fat along the length of the wound with a single movement. Multiple short incisions in this layer will produce a ragged wound with increased risk of bleeding and infection.

> Never push the blade of the scalpel where you cannot see what it is cutting unless you are 100% confident that no harm will result.

Scissors

The pair of scissors is a specialized piece of equipment. Get to understand how it works and become confident in its use with either hand. Most scissors are made for a right-handed action. If you are left-handed ask the theatre Sister if left-handed scissors are available, as it is less tiring to use the scissors designed for your dominant hand. The following description of how to use a right-handed pair of

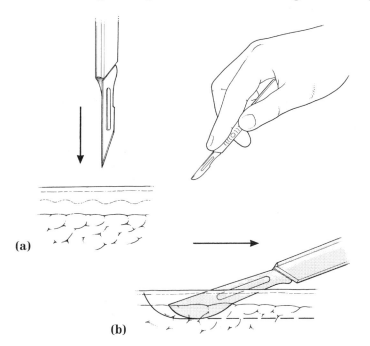

(a)

(b)

Fig. 1.6 **(a)** The straight-pointed blade is used for short stab incisions. **(b)** The curved blade is used for skin incision. The blade is pressed into the skin to the required depth and is then drawn along parallel to the surface. The shape of the blade ensures a smooth cut to the required depth.

scissors with either hand can be reversed to apply to a left-handed pair of scissors.

The action of the scissors depends on two movements (Fig. 1.7(a)).

The blades are brought together around a fulcrum so that the cutting edges overlap. In order for this cutting to be efficient, there must be close application of the two blades as they close. This is achieved partly by the inbuilt curvature (spring) of the blade and partly by the action of the surgeon. A correct action is particularly important to get the best out of a worn or loose pair of scissors.

Hold the scissors as if it is an extension of your index finger (Fig. 1.7(b)). Put your ring finger in one of the rings and rest the lateral margin of your thumb against the other ring. Steady the scissors with your index finger near the box joint. Your index finger can now control the tips of the scissors and the pressure of your thumb against the ring will act around the fulcrum of the joint to maintain apposition of the blades. Use the tips of the scissors for cutting whenever possible, as this makes full use of the spring in the blades and reduces the effect of a loose joint.

To use right-handed scissors with your left hand you will need to put your ring and index fingers as described above, but your thumb must now pass through the ring of the scissors in order to pull it towards the palm of your hand. This will help to maintain the correct motion around the fulcrum of the box joint and keep the blades in contact while they close.

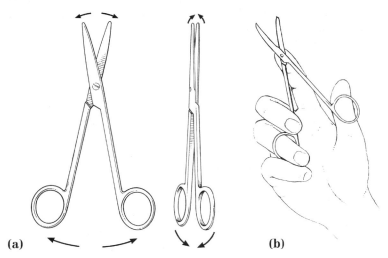

Fig. 1.7 Two movements are required for scissors to cut. The obvious movement around the joint to overlap the blades must be accompanied by a force designed to appose the two blades. This force is in a plane perpendicular to the closing movement of the scissors.

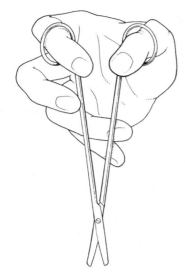

Fig. 1.8 A useful grip for working deep in a cavity with scissors. Apposition of the thumb keeps the blades working efficiently. The fingers hold one blade of the scissors while the thumb is used to control movement.

A more advanced grip, which is useful in situations where access into a deep incision is limited, is shown in Fig. 1.8.

Remember the principles by which the scissors function and maintain appropriate pressure with your thumb to appose the blades. Control the tips of the scissors with your fingers and make use of the wound edge to steady the blades if necessary.

Clips

Surgical clips have a ratchet mechanism between the handles to hold the clip closed when applied to a vessel or other tissues. Learn how to remove clips smoothly, without pulling at the tissue and without letting it go so quickly that the operator is unable to tighten the thread before the tissue retracts. Avoid turning your arm over to remove a clip and hold the instrument steady, as close as possible to the position in which it was applied.

When you are given a clip to hold while the surgeon ties a knot, look at the tip of the clip and note which way it curves. Check that there is a short length of clip projecting beyond the tissue to be tied. Hold the handles of the clip up slightly so that there is space between the clip and the patient for the surgeon to pass the thread behind it. When the surgeon has done this, lower the handles slightly to bring the tip of the clip away from contact with other parts of the wound.

This will enable the surgeon to put the thread safely and easily around the end of the clip. When the thread is round the end of the clip, rotate the instrument on its long axis to prevent the thread slipping off the clip before the knot is tied (Fig. 1.9).

As the knot tightens around the tissue, gently ease open the clip. This is a two-stage movement, the first stage being to push the handles apart in a plane perpendicular to the rings of the handles, while compressing the clip slightly to avoid it springing apart (Fig. 1.10).

The second movement is to open the blades smoothly to allow the thread to be tightened around the tissue. To do this with a clip in your right hand, hold the ring nearest to you between thumb and middle finger and apply pressure to the distant ring with your index finger. Raise this ring and pull it slightly towards you before allowing it to open with a controlled movement (Fig. 1.11). When opening a clip with your left hand hold the ring distant from you between your thumb and index finger and control the movement of the near ring with your middle finger.

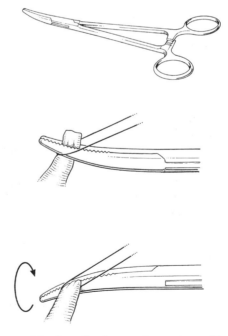

Fig. 1.9   Movement of the handles has an important effect on the curved tips of artery forceps. Use this to best advantage to expose the tips and then to prevent the thread from slipping while the knot is tied.

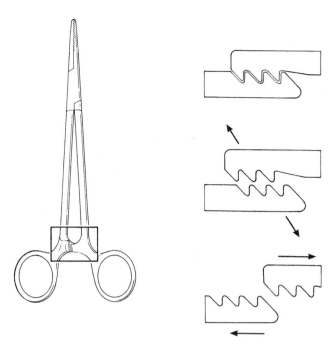

Fig. 1.10 Two movements are involved in opening a clip while a knot is tied. First, a perpendicular movement opens the ratchet while the clip is held closed. Second, the handles are gradually separated to open the tip of the clip.

Forceps

Surgical forceps should become second nature to you through constant use. You will normally hold them in your non-dominant hand to steady tissue while you cut with scissors or insert sutures. Get used to a variety of forceps and find which suit you best. Broad-toothed forceps allow a secure hold on the tissues with the least force applied per unit area of tissue grasped. Only use fine instruments if the tissues lie comfortably and no traction is required. Heavy forceps may be used for abdominal wall and abdominal skin closure. Softer forceps are suitable for handling bowel and blood vessels. Most specialists feel their own particular organ is 'special' – e.g. blood vessels, bile duct, ureter – and will tell you to avoid handling it with forceps if at all possible.

Hold the forceps between the thumb and index finger, resting on the middle finger (Fig. 1.12).

For particularly delicate work oppose the action of the thumb with both the index and middle fingers. This action is similar to using chopsticks. When suturing bowel or the vessels mentioned above, use

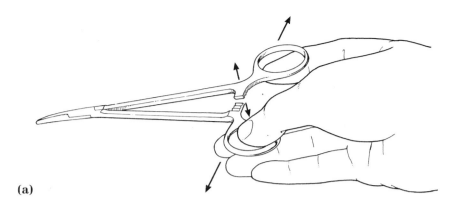

(a)

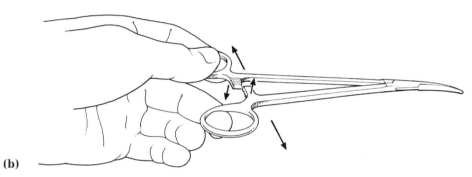

(b)

Fig. 1.11 **(a)** Hold the clip with your palm facing upwards, as described in the text. Upward movement of the index finger is followed by separation of the handles, with gradual release of the tips. **(b)** In a left-handed action the grip is reversed but the action is the same.

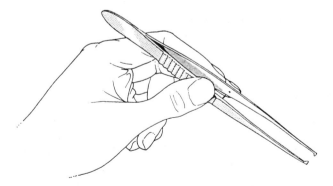

Fig. 1.12 Forceps should be held rather like chopsticks, with the action controlled between thumb and index finger.

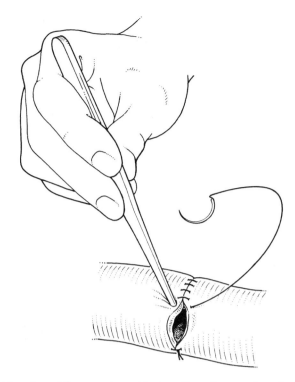

Fig. 1.13   Use closed forceps to guide together tissue edges in intestinal and vascular anastomosis.

the forceps to bring the edges of the tissue together, applying gentle pressure with the closed forceps near the suture if possible, in deference to the specialist prejudice already noted (Fig. 1.13). You can also use the closed tips of the forceps to guide the loop of a suture you are tightening, and to hold (gently!) the suture you have pulled through until your assistant can take it at the right tension.

DISSECTION TECHNIQUES

Incision of skin

Always use a knife to incise skin. The technique is described above (how to use the scalpel). If you use scissors to cut skin, firstly you will find it difficult and secondly you will crush the skin edges and impair wound healing. Some surgeons use diathermy to cut the skin but the power setting must be very high in order to avoid a burn of the skin edges. It is best to avoid this by using the knife.

Subcutaneous fat

When you are making an abdominal or thoracic incision it is necessary to divide the fatty tissue and fascial layer between the skin and the deep fascia. Many surgeons use a knife, as described above, which is quick but can produce troublesome bleeding. If you do use a knife, make a bold, firm sweep to produce a clean incised edge. Better, though, is the diathermy. Avoid needle diathermy because the needle point is dangerous and may stick in your finger. Use a spatula end on the diathermy which enables you to cut and coagulate with the same current. Get to know your own diathermy machine and adjust the power setting depending on the patient's build. The effect produced by the diathermy depends upon current density. Cutting diathermy is continuous and coagulation current is intermittent. Consequently the power used for coagulation is higher than for cutting. Very high current density with the coagulation current will still cut through the tissues. Apply the narrow edge of the spatula with firm pressure to the fat and cutting current. Increase the current density by reducing the area of contact. You can do this by using just the tip of the spatula. If you see a blood vessel, coagulate it by pressure with the broad face of the spatula without changing the current or power setting. If you have bleeding you can often stop the bleeding by pressure with the spatula while applying coagulation current. Alternatively, pick up bleeding points with a pair of insulated forceps and make contact between the metal of the forceps and the diathermy spatula. Do not use non-insulated metal forceps for this as there is a risk of short-circuiting through yourself, with a painful diathermy burn to your finger.

Division of fascia and muscle

When you have cut through the fat down to the fascia, the next step depends on whether you are cutting through a muscular area such as the chest or the right iliac fossa or whether you are making a midline incision in the abdomen. In the midline, use the knife or the diathermy on a cutting current to cut through the white fibrous tissue of linea alba. In the upper abdomen this will expose the fat of the falciform ligament. In the lower abdomen the fibrous tissue is less obvious, and you will come through on to fat and peritoneum between the muscle bellies. Incise peritoneum as described below.

When you are cutting through fascia with underlying muscle you will usually wish to divide both tissues in the line of the fascial and muscle fibres. Where the fascia is thin, such as external oblique in a gridiron incision or hernia repair, make a small incision in it with the knife and then extend the incision with scissors. Just open the tips of

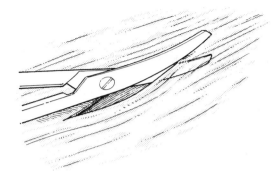

Fig. 1.14 When the fascia is exposed make a small excision in it and extend this by pushing the slightly opened blade of a pair of scissors along the line of the fibres. The scissors are held in a fixed position with the tips only slightly opened (inset).

the scissors, insert one blade beneath the fascia and push without closing the scissors in the line of the fibres (Fig. 1.14).

If you wish to open a muscle in the line of its fibres, make a small incision in the investing fascia, then insert the blades of the scissors between the fibres of the muscle. Open the blades, first in the line of the fibres then at right angles to this line, to separate the muscle. Immediately insert a Langenbeck retractor to hold back each edge of the separated muscle and if necessary extend the incision by lateral traction.

To divide these layers when you are cutting across the muscle, or for thoracotomy, it is better to use the diathermy. You may need to reduce the power setting after dividing the fat, particularly in obese patients. Aim to produce coagulation of the cut edge with simultaneous division of the tissue at the point of contact. Draw the spatula across the fascia to open it for the full length of the wound. Then divide the muscle progressively, working through the full depth of the muscle. Pick up any bleeding points with forceps and coagulate them as you go. By careful adjustment of the angle and length of contact between the diathermy spatula and the muscle you can achieve virtually bloodless muscle cutting incision.

It is unnecessary to elevate muscles over other instruments when dividing in this way with the diathermy. To do so merely risks short-circuit burns to the skin, and may displace the line of incision of the muscle away from the centre of the wound, making closure more difficult.

Specific manoeuvres to open the peritoneum and pleura and to close the abdomen and chest are described in the appropriate chapters.

HAEMOSTASIS

Careful haemostasis is essential in all branches of surgery. It is better to spot blood vessels before you divide them and either tie, clip or diathermy them as appropriate. If bleeding occurs try to pick up just the bleeding point and not surrounding tissue. If you include too much tissue in the diathermy forceps there will be low current density and poor coagulation. A tie placed around a large bunch of soft tissue is more likely to slip than one placed around the vessel alone.

Clips

If you identify a vessel before you divide it, place the clip so that its tip projects 1 mm beyond the vessel. Check as you close the clip that the points are not catching any other tissue. This slight projection will enable you to tie securely beneath the clip.

DIATHERMY

Monopolar diathermy

Pick up the smallest amount of tissue needed to control the bleeding point. Ideally this should be the vessel alone. Apply current until the vessel is coagulated. You may see the blood within it turn white, and you will know that is sufficient. It is not necessary and may be harmful to produce large amounts of black charred tissue around the bleeding point. Do not let the tips project beyond the tissue to be coagulated: this may damage adjacent tissue unnecessarily.

Bipolar diathermy

This achieves coagulation by current passing between the two blades of the forceps. It provides precise, localized coagulation without exposing the whole patient to an electric current. It is especially useful in patients fitted with pacemakers.

Pick up only the tissue to be coagulated. Do not press too hard on the forceps as this will short-circuit the current and lead to failure of coagulation. There will be less visible evidence of tissue destruction when effective coagulation has been achieved. Do not prolong coagulation in order to destroy surrounding tissue.

Suture ligation

When there is bleeding that is difficult to identify, or the tissues are very soft, it is best to stop the bleeding with a stitch. In order to do this you need to compress the tissue all around the bleeding point and a single bite with the needle is not sufficient. Use a Z stitch, taking a bite at least 1 cm deep and 1 cm wide on each side of the bleeding point (Fig. 1.15).

Pass the needle on one side of the bleeding point and draw the suture through, leaving sufficient length to tie. Hold the two ends of

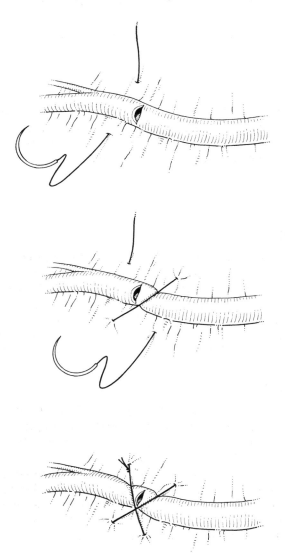

Fig. 1.15 Suture ligation of a bleeding point. Two passes of the needle are required, one on each side of the bleeding point, to ensure ligation of the vessel either side of the injury. The track of the needle describes a letter Z. When tied the suture resembles a letter X.

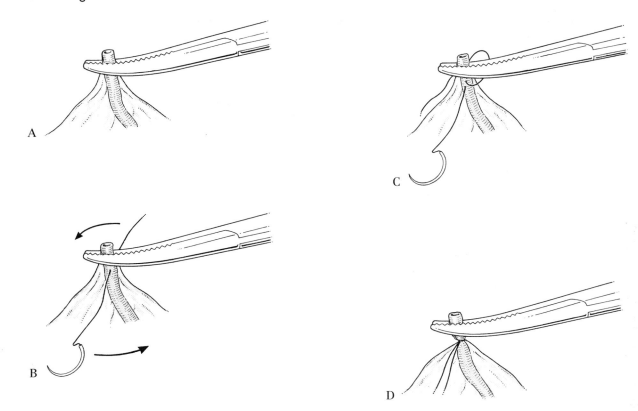

Fig. 1.16 Two passes of the needle through the pedicle are required to ensure that the thread completely encircles the pedicle before the clip is removed. Take care to pass the loose end and the needle end around opposite sides of the pedicle.

the stitch to begin control of the bleeding and carefully make a corresponding bite on the other side of the bleeding point (Fig. 1.15). Pull the stitch tight and tie a knot over the bleeding point. If correctly placed this will invariably stop the bleeding.

Suture ligation of vessels

Sometimes to get secure control of a large vessel it is better to use a suture, as a tie may roll off. This is appropriate for a wide cystic duct, and for the splenic artery after splenectomy, for example. Pass the needle of a 2/0 Vicryl suture through the vessel below the clip. Leave the end of the stitch long enough to tie comfortably and pass this end around the tips of the forceps. Mount the needle again, and take it behind the clip to pass it through the pedicle a second time, close to the first pass. Tie the stitch below the tip of the clip. This minimizes the contortions required of your assistant who is holding the clip. You have now completely encircled the vessel and anchored the tie in the vessel (Fig. 1.16).

ISOLATION OF NERVES AND VESSELS

Longitudinal structures such as nerves and vessels can be isolated by separating them from surrounding structures, passing a curved in-

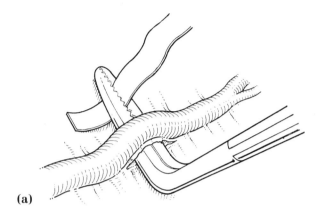

(a)

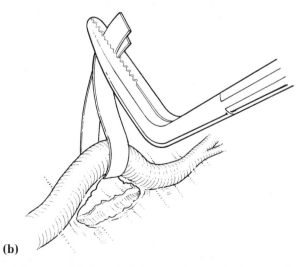

(b)

Fig. 1.17 **(a)** Pass a right-angled forceps beneath the vessel or nerve and open the tips. **(b)** Grasp the thread or tape in the jaws of the forceps and withdraw it to elevate the structure.

strument beneath and drawing a thread or tape around the structure to elevate it from the surrounding tissue (Fig. 1.17).

If the structure is beneath an investing layer of fascia, incise the fascia lateral to and parallel to the nerve or vessel and pass a right-angled forceps such as a Lahey behind it. Adjust the angle of the Lahey to bring the points up, raising the fascia on the opposite side, and open the points of the Lahey slightly. Incise this tissue and close the points to allow them to appear through the fascia. Only when you can clearly see clean metal should you then increase the distance between the tips of the Lahey to mobilize a length of nerve or vessel.

In general, arteries and veins can be dissected close on their surface. Veins are very loosely attached to surrounding tissue and can easily be cleaned once the shiny purplish surface of the vein has been reached (Chapter 13). Arteries are best dissected very close to the adventitia. Carefully come down through the surrounding connective tissue and lymphatics (diathermy lymphatic vessels to seal them) until you reach a plane on the adventitia. Dissect carefully around this very close to the vessel and you will find that the artery will be easily freed from the surrounding lymphatics and areolar tissue. Again, a Lahey forceps or other right-angled forceps can be passed close to the vessel; when you have identified the tips on the far side of the vessel, develop the plane close to the wall of the artery.

When you have isolated the structure by passing a clip behind it, place an atraumatic sling (usually a Silastic strip or a soft thread), around the vessel by grasping one end of the sling in the forceps and drawing it behind the vessel. If appropriate, tie the thread securely and ask yourself whether you need to apply two ties (usually a wise precaution on large vessels).

> Allow a safety margin of connective tissue with its supporting blood vessel when dissecting nerves and ureter.

> When going round a vein, make sure you can see the plane of dissection on both sides of the vessel. It is very easy to lift up the vein wall behind and tear or cut it. Do not apply any force unless you can clearly see the metal tips of the clip.

SUTURING DRAINS

Use a braided suture such as silk to secure drains. Pass the needle through the skin close to the drain exit site, then tie a reef knot to leave a small loop of suture anchored in the skin. This knot will serve as a fixed point to tie against (Fig. 1.18).

Tie the suture around the drain so the threads pass perpendicular to the long axis. This will ensure the tie is around the shortest circumference. Take another turn around the drain with each end of the thread and tie it again. Avoid taking the threads along the drain to produce a 'zig zag' appearance. If the suture begins to slip it will immediately slacken and the drain can then fall out (Fig. 1.18).

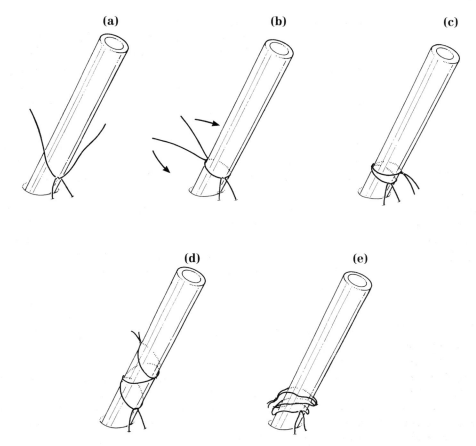

Fig. 1.18 **(a)** Tie a reef knot in the suture 5–10 mm from the skin. **(b)** Pass the ties around the drain and fix them securely with a reef knot. **(c)** Pass each end once round a drain and tie them again. **(d)** Avoid a 'gaiter' effect, which will easily loosen.

TWIST DRAINS

To make a small capillary drain for a subcutaneous cavity such as that left by excision of a lipoma or a breast lump, take a length of 0 nylon and attach an artery forceps to its midpoint. Attach another clip to both ends and twist the double strands by turning the clips in opposite directions (Fig. 1.19).

Keep tension on the two clips to prevent the thread tangling, and ask your assistant to apply a third clip at the midpoint of the twisted strands. Gradually allow the two clips at each end to move together, as you continue to rotate them and the third clip will drop down, creating a four-stranded twist (Fig. 1.19). When all the suture ma-

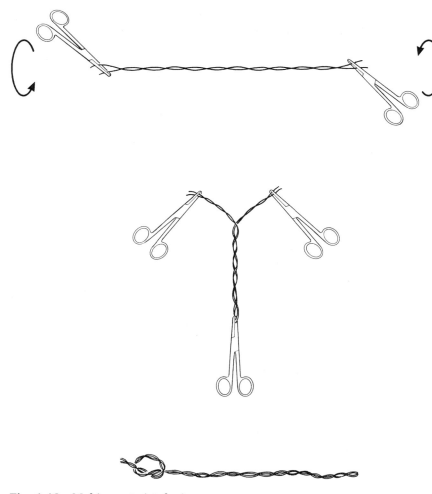

Fig. 1.19 Making a twist drain.

terial has been taken up in the four-stranded twist, grasp this end firmly and tie a single throw to prevent it coming undone.

Use this drain by placing it through the suture line, with the loop in the cavity and the knot outside. This will allow exudate and blood to seep out into the dressing, and it is easily removed the day after the operation.

SKIN CLOSURE

The aim of skin closure is to produce accurate apposition of the wound edges, in all layers of the skin, and with minimal dead space beneath. On the limbs, face and breasts it is generally necessary to use stitches that penetrate the skin. On the neck and trunk and in the groins, a subcuticular suture will often do the job and is less likely to become infected. Slight eversion is thought to be beneficial, as subsequent scar contracture will not then produce a dimple.

Simple skin sutures

This suture (Fig. 1.20) should bring together the deep layers of the skin, but you should not aim to obliterate all the dead space beneath if there is a deep wound. (If necessary use a few sutures to close the dead space.)

   Pass the needle through the skin, starting perpendicular to the surface and arcing round to cross the wound just below the dermis. Complete the suture with the mirror image, passing from just below the dermis to leave the skin perpendicular to its surface. Tie the suture with the knot to one side, so that it does not become incorporated in coagulum over the wound. This stitch can be run as a continuous suture in the form of a blanket stitch, which looks very neat.

Mattress suture

The mattress stitch aims to close the deep part of the wound, to obliterate dead space and to slightly evert the skin edges. It is particularly useful if interrupted simple sutures are beginning to cause inversion of the wound edges. Start at least 1 cm from the wound edge and go deeply into the wound as far as practical. If the wound

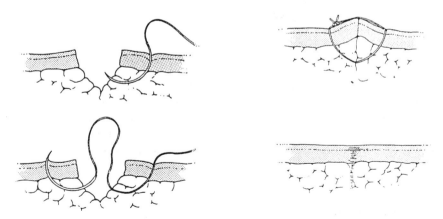

Fig. 1.20 Skin stitches take only the skin and small amount of subcutaneous tissue. The tension in the stitch should be adjusted to produce slight eversion.

edge is undermined, pass perpendicularly through the full thickness of the wound edge. Pull the stitch through and bring the needle out in the corresponding fashion on the opposite side of the wound, leaving the skin perpendicularly. Next pick up just the skin edge about 1 mm from the cut surface and bring the needle point through the dermis. Come out of the wound on the opposite side in a similar way and then tie the stitch with the knot over the original entry point (Fig. 1.21).

Subcuticular suture

This technique has many advantages, as it is less prone to infection and gives a better scar. Absorbable suture material does not require removal, but may produce an angry red reaction in the scar. Monofilament non-absorbable suture material requires removal, but produces no reaction. Use polypropylene, which has very low drag and is less difficult to remove.

Enter the skin about 1 cm from the end of the incision, using a straight needle. Start with the wound edge nearest to your right hand and closest to you. Pass the needle beneath the skin in the dermis and bring the point out in the wound. Pick up one side of the wound for 8–10 mm; keep the needle parallel with the skin surface in the dermis. Repeat this on the other side, entering the skin at a point opposite or only just behind the exit point on the opposite side (Fig. 1.22). If you go too far back on each side it will take longer to place the suture and it will be much harder to remove.

If the wound is more than 12 cm long, bring the suture over the wound at a convenient point. In very long wounds you may need two or more skin loops. These should be no more than 10 cm apart. After exiting the skin at one wound edge, enter the opposite edge at the same level but bring the needle out perpendicular to the wound for 1 cm before coming out through the skin. Re-enter the dermis on the opposite side at the same level on the wound, so that this suture when pulled through will lie perpendicular to the line of the incision. Bring the needle point out at an appropriate place to begin the subcuticular suture once again.

If your consultant wishes you to use an absorbable suture for subcuticular stitch, you can place Dexon or (colourless) Vicryl without tying a knot. If you are operating under local anaesthetic, remember to bring the needle through the skin within an anaesthetized area! Make three passes in the shape of a Z or triangle, ensuring that the suture runs in the dermis with each pass. The drag of the suture in the dermis, combined with the angles at each entry point, will stop it slipping through. You must be careful to pull through sufficient length of suture material with the first pass, as you will not be able

When applying a subcuticular suture, do not pull the full length of the stitch through every time. Leave a loop outside the skin and pull through every 5 cm or so for absorbable sutures. For non-absorbables pull the full length through only when you have finished, or each time you make a skin loop (Fig. 1.22).

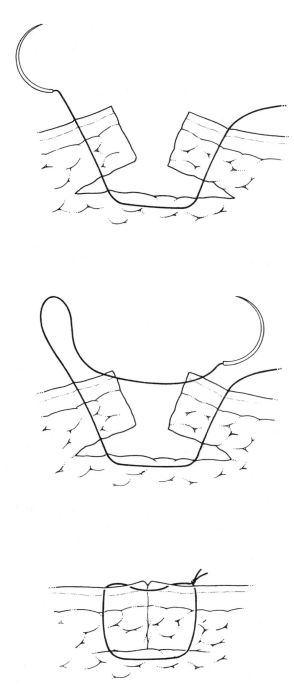

Fig. 1.21 Mattress suture. This stitch apposes the deeper layers and everts the skin.

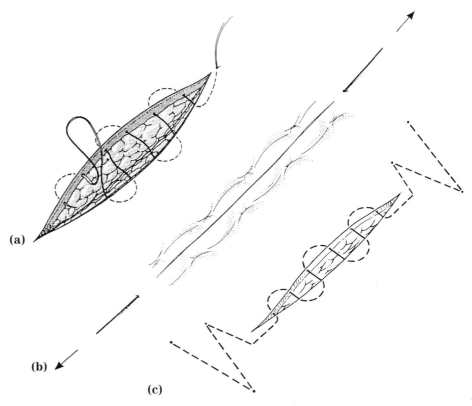

(a)

(b)

(c)

Fig. 1.22 Subcuticular suture. **(a)** Place the needle through the subcuticular layer and dermis, and advance along the wound in a regular step-wise fashion. Do not double back. **(b)** Regular progression ensures good apposition of the wound edges when this stitch is pulled straight. **(c)** Subcuticular absorbable sutures can be fixed by three passes in the dermis at each end of the wound.

to correct the length at the end. Repeat the procedure at the end of the incision and then cut off both ends flush with the skin. This is a secure closure that avoids problems with knots in the superficial layers of the skin.

CYTOLOGY AND BIOPSY

Fine needle aspiration

Indication

Aspiration cytology is useful for the diagnosis of any subcutaneous lump, particularly lymph nodes to differentiate metastatic tumour from lymphoma, and for breast lumps. Thyroid nodules and other swellings in the neck may also be biopsied but this should be carried out under supervision.

To obtain a sample for cytology from a solid lesion you will need a 20 ml syringe, a green (21 gauge) needle, and some microscope slides.

Place the patient comfortably on a couch, with the lump exposed and the area relaxed. Fit the needle on the syringe and move the plunger in and out to make sure it is not stuck and to empty the barrel of air.

Hold the lesion between the finger and thumb of one hand, with the syringe in the other. Direct the needle along the shortest path through the skin into the centre of the lump. Now, apply suction to the needle and move it backwards and forwards within the lump (Fig. 1.23). Release the suction on the syringe before you remove the needle from the lump.

Withdraw the needle and syringe intact, remove the syringe from the needle and half fill it with air. Re-attach the needle and squirt the contained material on to a microscope slide. If there is copious material, spread it on to two or more slides.

> The aim is to fill the needle with cellular material. Make sure the vacuum in the syringe has been fully relaxed before you remove the needle, to avoid the aspirated tissue being sucked into the syringe.

Needle biopsy

This differs from aspiration cytology in that a core of tissue can be removed for histology. Needle biopsy is generally more uncomfortable for the patient than aspiration. It may be useful for lesions in the breast or the prostate and for the preoperative diagnosis of soft-tissue masses in the limbs. Lymph nodes are best removed by excision biopsy to obtain an accurate histological diagnosis.

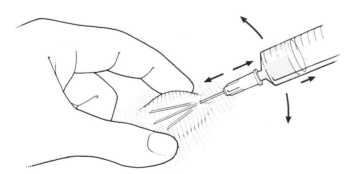

Fig. 1.23   Fine-needle aspiration for cytology. Hold the lesion between the index finger and thumb of one hand and move the needle in and out in different directions while maintaining suction on the syringe.

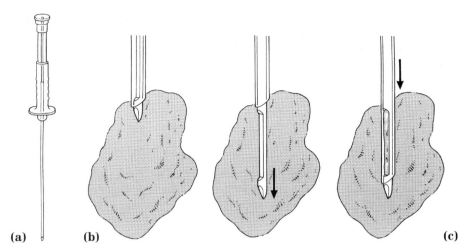

(a)   **(b)**   **(c)**

Fig. 1.24 The biopsy needle has an outer cover, which can take in the cut-away section of the inner needle. **(b)** The tissue to be biopsied prolapses into the cut-away. **(c)** The outer sleeve is advanced to enclose a core of tissue, which is removed within the needle.

Biopsy needles

There is a range of biopsy needles. One is illustrated. The Tru-cut® needle consists of a hollow needle with an obturator. The obturator has a 'cut-away' which can be advanced beyond the outer sleeve (Fig. 1.24).

When the cut-away section is exposed the tissue prolapses into it and the sleeve is then advanced over this section to enclose a core of tissue.

Technique

Anaesthetize the skin with 1% lignocaine. Make a small incision with a No. 11 blade over the lesion. Insert the needle through this incision and advance it in the closed position up to the edge of the lesion. Next advance the inner needle into the lesion until the cut-away is fully exposed. Then hold the central needle steady and advance the outer sleeve over it to enclose the core of tissue. Ensure that the outer sleeve is fully pushed home, rotate the needle through 90° and then withdraw it. If necessary apply some gentle pressure to stop any bleeding.

Open the needle to inspect the core of removed tissue. In general, tumours are hard and white and subcutaneous fat is yellow and soft. If you are not sure you have obtained a good sample, make one more pass with the needle. Remove the core from the needle by laying the needle on a piece of filter paper, to which the core will adhere. Gently slide the needle away from the tissue, then place the sample into formol saline.

Local anaesthetic techniques

Andrew J. T. Sansome and J. Knighton

Local anaesthetics are chemical compounds that reversibly inhibit the transmission of peripheral nerves impulses. They are classified according to their chemical structure into esters (cocaine and procaine) or amides (most of the modern local anaesthetics, including lignocaine, prilocaine and bupivacaine; Fig. 2.1).

Their common mode of action is to block nerve axon sodium channels, preventing depolarization and propagation of the action potential. Their different physicochemical properties confer different rates of onset, duration of action and potency on the individual agents, as outlined below.

Local anaesthetic toxicity

When local anaesthetic agents are used great care should be taken to avoid toxicity. The esters may produce a profound systemic allergic reaction that is dose-independent, while the more commonly used amides produce dose-dependent systemic toxicity whose severity depends on the plasma concentration achieved. The dose of drug administered must therefore be restricted, especially in highly vascular areas, where systemic absorption is rapid. Great care must be taken (by repeated aspiration) to avoid intravenous injection. The safe maximum doses commonly quoted are displayed in Table 2.1; though generally accepted, these are only guidelines since the safe dose varies considerably between patients and depends on the site of administration, rate of absorption, pattern of distribution to other organs, and the rate of metabolism and excretion. Of all the factors that contribute to the risk of toxicity, the dose of the drug and the site of injection are the most important.

The combination of lignocaine or prilocaine with a vasoconstrictor such as 1:200000 adrenaline reduces the rate of systemic absorption, increases the duration of action and reduces the risk of dose-dependent toxicity. This allows the maximum dose of 0.5% lignocaine with adrenaline to be increased to 7 mg/kg.

Systemic toxicity is similar for all agents, resulting in numbness

Table 2.1   Maximum 'safe' dose of commonly used local anaesthetics

Lignocaine	3 mg/kg (for a 70 kg man = 21 ml of 1%)
Bupivacaine	2 mg/kg (for a 70 kg man = 28 ml of 0.5%)
Prilocaine	6 mg/kg (for a 70 kg man = 42 ml of 1%)

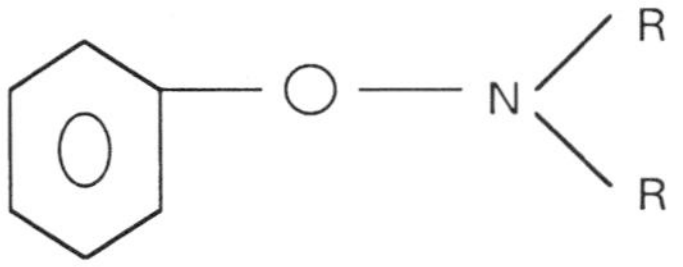

Aromatic ring   Amide or ester   Amine and hydrocarbon groups

link

Fig. 2.1   General structure of the local anaesthetics.

Table 2.2   Local anaesthetic toxic reactions

Overdose level	Features likely	Action taken
Mild to moderate	Metallic taste Talkativeness Visual, auditory disturbance Excitability Slurred speech Tremor and generalized twitching Tachycardia Tachypnoea Hypertension	**Stop injection** Call experienced help Adequate i.v. access Supplementary oxygen ECG, BP and pulse oximetry monitoring Supportive treatment as below, if required **Explain** and **reassure patient**
Moderate to severe	Tonic-clonic seizures Generalized CNS depression Hypotension, bradycardia Cardiovascular collapse Respiratory arrest **May be rapid progression to CVS and RS collapse**	**Stop injection** **Call anaesthetic help** **'A, B, C' resuscitation** Intubation and ventilation Rapid i.v. volume expansion Atropine, adrenaline as necessary Control fitting with i.v. diazepam or thiopentone Transfer to ICU Continue full support until levels have fallen

Note: In bupivacaine toxicity treatment may be difficult and therefore cardiorespiratory resuscitation should be prolonged and tingling, especially of the tongue and mouth, followed by tinnitus, blurred vision, restlessness, drowsiness and muscular twitching as higher blood levels are reached. Ultimately, there is progression to convulsions, coma and cardiorespiratory arrest, leading to death.

When performing any regional anaesthetic technique or local nerve block, the provision of patient monitoring adequate to detect the development of toxicity is mandatory; full resuscitation facilities must be available and the 'operator' must be appropriately trained. All but the most simple local blocks should be performed and monitored by a second operator. Should any evidence of systemic toxicity be identified, stop the injection of local anaesthetic and the procedure. Seek the help of senior anaesthetic staff urgently (Table 2.2).

Choice of local anaesthetic agent

For most purposes the three most commonly used agents, lignocaine, bupivacaine and prilocaine, will suffice. Most agents are compared to **lignocaine** (used as 1% or 2% concentrations), which has a rapid onset of action and is potent but has a limited duration of action.

Prilocaine (concentrations 0.5% and 1%) has an onset and duration of action similar to lignocaine but is considerably less toxic in large doses and is therefore the agent of choice in blocks requiring large volumes of local anaesthetic. It is the only agent widely used for intravenous regional anaesthesia (IVRA; Bier's block) in the UK.

Bupivacaine (concentrations 0.25% and 0.5%) is a highly potent local anaesthetic with a duration of action approaching twice that of lignocaine but with a slower onset. It carries a greater likelihood of systemic toxicity than either of the other agents, and may have direct cardiac effects. It is contraindicated for IVRA and should be avoided in blocks requiring large volumes of local anaesthetic, but is ideal for local infiltration to provide postoperative analgesia.

WOUND INFILTRATION

Use local anaesthetics by infiltration to provide anaesthesia or analgesia during and/or after surgical procedures, e.g. inguinal hernia repair, wound exploration, superficial suturing. This is useful as either the sole anaesthetic technique or as an adjunct to general anaesthesia.

Bupivacaine 0.2% is the most useful agent, providing analgesia for around 3 hours following local infiltration; this may be increased to 5–6 hours if the combination with 1:200000 adrenaline is used.

Lignocaine 1% or 2% will provide analgesia for around 2 hours when plain solutions are used or 4 hours when combined with 1:200000 adrenaline.

Care should be taken to avoid intravascular injection and to prevent the administration of potentially toxic doses of the drug, as detailed above.

Skin infiltration

Infiltrating local anaesthetic into the skin allows you to perform minor operations on the skin or subcutaneous tissues. Use a fine gauge needle such as 25 gauge on the syringe and insert it into the skin. The needle should be just deep to the dermis and a 'bleb' should be visible during infiltration. (N. B. The nerve endings lie in the skin layer rather than the subcutaneous tissues.)

Infiltrating sensitive areas

The palm of the hand and sole of the feet are particularly sensitive and direct puncture of these areas can be avoided even if the palm or sole needs to be anaesthetized. In these circumstances, place the fingertips of the left hand on the area of palm or sole to be anaesthetized and insert the needle through the dorsal surface of the hand or foot (Fig. 2.2).

Avoid the metacarpals (tarsals) and pass the needle towards the left fingertips. As soon as you feel the needle tip tent the palmar skin, begin gentle infiltration. Withdraw and reinsert the needle to adjacent areas until the area of concern is infiltrated.

Digital nerve blocks

Indication

Digital nerve block should not be performed when there is any possibility of distal ischaemia. Local anaesthetic solutions containing vasoconstrictors must never be used.

This highly effective block of the fingers or toes may be used to provide anaesthesia for minor surgery and analgesia postoperatively or following trauma.

Technique

The fingers and toes are innervated by dorsal and ventral branches both medially and laterally.

Both 1–2% plain lignocaine and 0.5% plain bupivacaine are suitable. The latter provides a block of longer duration, lasting up to 12 hours, and is therefore probably the agent of choice.

Place the patient's hand palm down with your left index or middle finger beneath the proximal phalanx of the digit to be blocked.

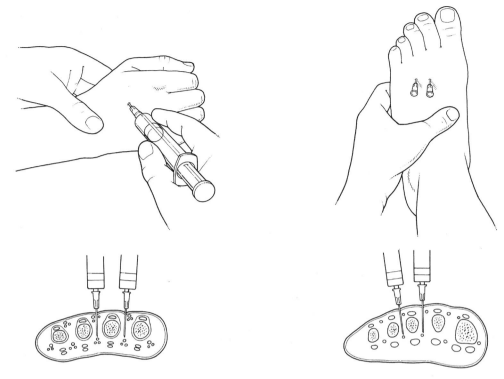

Fig. 2.2   Technique for infiltration of the palm and sole.

Introduce a 23 gauge needle into the dorsolateral aspect of the digit and as it is advanced inject 1–2 ml of local anaesthetic (Fig. 2.3).

Stop injecting when pressure is felt by the palpating finger. Repeat the procedure on the other side of the digit to produce a bilateral block.

Penile block

Indications

This relatively simple block may be used for circumcision, meatotomy or dorsal slit. It avoids the bladder dysfunction and motor blockade that may accompany caudal anaesthesia and provides equivalent analgesia for localized procedures.

Technique

The sensory supply of the penis is largely derived from the dorsal nerves (S2, 3, 4), while the base is innervated by the genital branch of the genitofemoral nerve (L1).

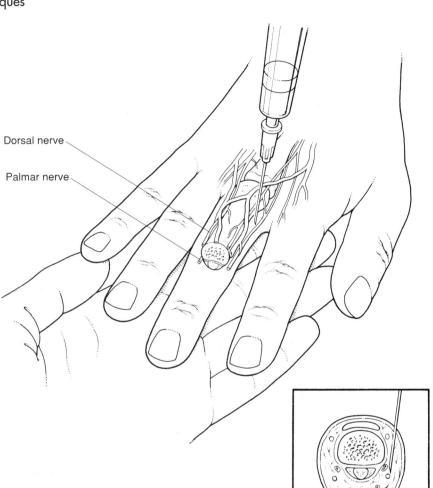

Dorsal nerve

Palmar nerve

Fig. 2.3 Digital nerve block: note the position of the dorsal and palmar nerves.

Use either 0.5% plain bupivacaine or 1% plain lignocaine.

Place the patient supine and a finger in the midline below the symphysis pubis. Raise a skin weal and introduce a 23 gauge needle in the midline. Advance directly dorsally to a depth of 3–4 cm (immediately superficial to the corpora cavernosa) and infiltrate 5–10 ml of local anaesthetic (Fig. 2.4(a)).

Infiltrate a further 5–10 ml of local anaesthetic solution subcutaneously around the base of the penis, which will block the genital

> Local anaesthetic solutions containing vasoconstrictors must never be used. Great care must be taken to avoid intravascular injection.

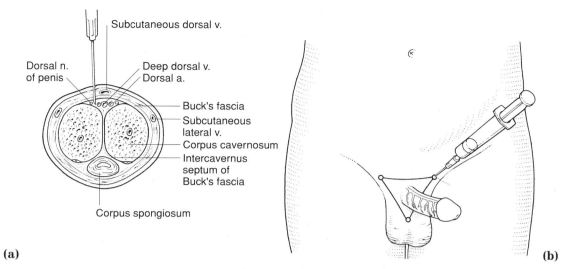

Fig. 2.4 **(a)** Technique of penile nerve block. **(b)** Subcutaneous infiltration to block the branches of the genitofemoral nerve. a. = artery; v. = vein; n. = nerve.

branches of the genitofemoral-femoral nerve and provide a much better block (Fig. 2.4(b); see also Chapter 12).

Field block for inguinal hernia repair

Indications

The field block may be used either in conjunction with general anaesthesia, when it will provide excellent postoperative analgesia, or alone as the sole anaesthetic technique. It is indicated in patients who are considered unfit for general anaesthesia or in whom it is wished to minimize the perioperative administration of opiates.

Anatomy

The musculocutaneous innervation of the groin is derived from the ventral primary rami of T11 and T12 (subcostal nerve), together with the ilioinguinal (L1) and iliohypogastric (L1) branches of the lumbar plexus (Fig. 2.5).

The subcostal nerve, after leaving the 12th rib, runs between transversus and internal oblique and becomes superficial to supply the skin over the lower end of the rectus sheath. The anterior cutaneous branch of the iliohypogastric nerve starts between transversus and internal oblique but penetrates the latter 2 cm medial to the anterior superior iliac spine (ASIS) to run deep to external oblique.

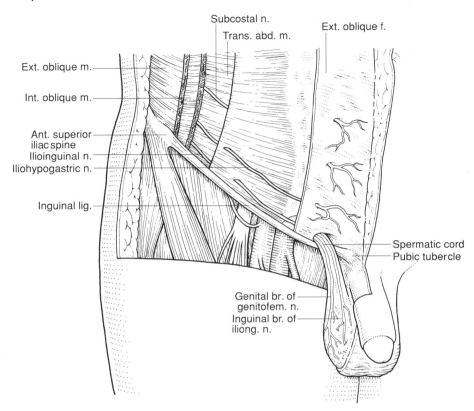

Fig. 2.5 Nerve supply of the inguinal region. m. = muscle; n. = nerve.

About 2–3 cm above the superficial ring it penetrates external oblique and supplies the skin over the medial groin and symphysis pubis. The ilioinguinal nerve penetrates internal oblique a little more medially, traverses the inguinal canal and emerges through either the external ring or external oblique fascia to supply the skin of the scrotum and adjacent thigh. The lateral part of the inguinal ligament is supplied by the lateral cutaneous branches of the subcostal and iliohypogastric nerves, which penetrate internal oblique lateral to the ASIS. The genital branch of the genitofemoral-femoral nerve also runs in the inguinal canal and supplies a branch to the medial end of the groin.

Technique

To provide sufficient anaesthesia to permit inguinal herniorrhaphy, large volumes (approx. 40–50 ml) of local anaesthetic are required, and therefore care must be taken to avoid the administration of potentially toxic doses. Bupivacaine 0.25% or prilocaine 0.5–1%, in both cases with or without 1:200 000 adrenaline, are suitable.

Since the principal nerves supplying the groin all lie close together anteromedial to the anterior superior iliac spine between the muscle layers, they may be conveniently blocked at this site.

With the patient placed supine, introduce a long 22 gauge short-bevel needle from a point 3 cm medial to the anterior superior iliac spine and direct it slightly laterally, down towards the ilium. Inject approximately 10 ml of local anaesthetic through the full thickness of the muscle layers (lateral cutaneous branches of the subcostal and iliohypogastric nerves). As the individual muscle layers are traversed you should feel a distinct loss of resistance or 'click'. From the same site, infiltrate approximately 15 ml of local anaesthetic in a mediocaudal direction immediately deep to the external oblique aponeurosis in a fan-shaped pattern (iliohypogastric and ilioinguinal

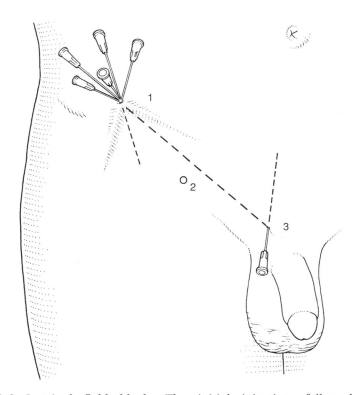

Fig. 2.6 Inguinal field block. The initial injection, followed by a mediocaudal fan, is made from point 1. The genital branch of the genitofemoral nerve, N, is blocked at point 2 and a midline band infiltration is made at point 3. Finally, the line of the incision (dotted) is infiltrated.

nerves). Introduce the needle perpendicular to the skin at a point 3 cm above the junction of the medial and middle third of the inguinal ligament and deposit a further 5–10 ml of local anaesthetic just deep to external oblique (genital branch of genitofemoral-femoral nerve; Fig. 2.6).

Introduce the needle immediately rostral to the pubic tubercle and infiltrate 5–10 ml of local anaesthetic subcutaneously in a cephalad direction (fibres crossing over from the other side). Finally, infiltrate the line of the incision subcutaneously with a further 5–10 ml. Once exposed it may be necessary to infiltrate the neck of the peritoneal sack (5 ml).

The block requires 15–30 minutes to become fully effective, particularly when 0.25% bupivacaine is used.

> Use a 19 gauge needle to perforate the skin before inserting the block needle.

Femoral nerve block

Indications

Although supplying sensation to only part of the lower limb, a femoral nerve block is a useful technique. It will provide good analgesia for fractures of the proximal third of the femoral shaft, is useful for anterior knee surgery and will permit the majority of varicose vein surgery. In combination with a block of the lateral cutaneous nerve, it provides anaesthesia for the collection of split skin grafts from the thigh.

The femoral nerve may be blocked alone or in combination with the lateral cutaneous nerve of the thigh and the obturator nerves in a 'three in one' block.

Anatomy

The femoral nerve (L2, 3, 4) leaves the pelvis beneath the inguinal ligament, lying on the psoas muscle, slightly behind and lateral to the fascial sheath that contains the femoral artery and vein. The proximity of the femoral nerve to the sheath may vary, such that its relation to the femoral artery is an inconsistent landmark. The femoral nerve, *via* its anterior and posterior divisions, supplies the hip and knee joint and the skin of the medial leg and anterior thigh (Fig. 2.7).

Technique

A quantity of 10–20 ml of 1% plain lignocaine or prilocaine or 0.5% plain bupivacaine is suitable for femoral nerve block. Three in one block requires 30 ml of 1% plain lignocaine or prilocaine or 0.375% plain bupivacaine. Great care should be taken with solutions containing adrenaline because of the risk of intravascular injection.

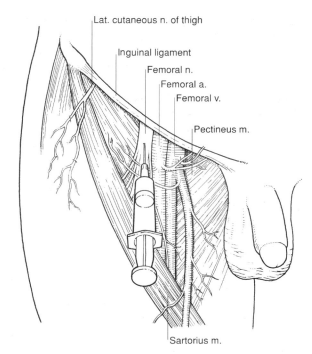

Lat. cutaneous n. of thigh

Inguinal ligament

Femoral n.

Femoral a.

Femoral v.

Pectineus m.

Sartorius m.

Fig. 2.7   Femoral nerve block. Note the needle position and angulation. a. = artery; v. = vein; m. = muscle; n. = nerve.

Femoral nerve   With the patient supine, identify the pubic tubercle and anterior superior iliac spine and palpate the femoral artery at the midpoint of the inguinal ligament. Introduce a 22 gauge short-bevel needle approximately 1 cm lateral to the artery, direct it crani-ally at an angle of 45° to the skin (a click should be felt as the fascia lata is penetrated) and advance to a depth of 3–4 cm (Fig. 2.7). If paraesthesia is elicited, inject 10 ml of local anaesthetic; if not, with-draw the needle and redirect it more laterally. If the nerve cannot be identified, 20 ml of local anaesthetic is infiltrated in a fan pattern lateral to the artery, to a depth of 4 cm.

'Three in one'   Since the obturator, lateral cutaneous and femoral nerves all arise from the lumbar plexus and lie in a common myofascial plane, a large volume of local anaesthetic introduced around the latter will spread to affect all three. Paraesthesia must be sought, as above, and once the correct position is determined the needle must be held still. Apply pressure just distal to the injection site to encourage the proximal spread of 30 ml of local anaesthetic.

The block may take some 15–20 minutes to become established.

> Use a short, flexible connection between the syringe and needle to minimize the risk of displacement during the injection.

IVRA (Bier's block)

Indications

This is a safe and excellent block provided that correct technique is observed. It provides very good analgesia for any short (less than 1 hour) procedure on the forearm or lower leg, including manipulation of fractures, carpal tunnel decompression and other minor surgery to the hand and foot. It provides good muscle relaxation in the majority of patients and the use of a tourniquet (with exsanguination) guarantees a bloodless surgical field.

Contraindications

Conditions where the use of a tourniquet may risk ischaemic damage (e.g. sickle cell disease, Raynaud's disease or scleroderma) are absolute contraindications, as is a history of local anaesthetic sensitivity, untreated heart block or severe cardiovascular disease, because of the risk of local anaesthetic toxicity.

Bier's block is not suitable for children under 10 years old, who may have highly vascular long bones, rendering a tourniquet ineffective.

Fatalities have occurred with this technique when bupivacaine has been used, because of its direct cardiac toxicity, and use of this drug is therefore never indicated for Bier's block.

Technique

Bupivacaine, even in low concentrations, should not be used for this technique. Local anaesthetic solutions containing vasoconstrictors must also not be used.

Using 0.5% prilocaine, a block of the upper limb requires a volume of 40 ml, while the lower leg needs 60 ml.

Patients must be fasted as for general anaesthesia and there should be two trained doctors present (one as operator and one as anaesthetist). Appropriate monitoring and resuscitation facilities must be available. Insert an intravenous cannula distally in the arm to be anaesthetized and another in another limb, in order to permit the management of an adverse reaction.

A double-cuffed pneumatic tourniquet is placed around the upper arm and the limb is then exsanguinated, either by elevation for 3 minutes or by the use of an Esmarch bandage, The proximal tourniquet is inflated to 100 mmHg above systolic arterial blood pressure (and a check is made that distal pulses have been abolished). Slowly inject local anaesthetic solution over 2 minutes and the isolated arm will be seen to discolour. Discomfort from the tourniquet will be alleviated if after 5–10 minutes the distal cuff is inflated and, once you are satisfied that the pressure in this also exceeds the systolic blood pressure by 100 mmHg, deflate the proximal cuff. Anaesthesia is usually established within 10 minutes.

The tourniquet should not be deflated for at least 15 minutes, irrespective of the duration of the operation. ECG and blood pressure monitoring are mandatory during the procedure, and should be continued for 5 minutes after final cuff deflation. Bilateral blocks may be used but should not be performed simultaneously.

> Do not exceed the maximum safe dose of local anaesthetic.

Complications

With good technique and suitable equipment, complications are rare. Methaemoglobinaemia may occur if more than 600 mg of prilocaine is used, and the onset of tinnitus, dizziness, convulsions or cardiovascular instability should immediately raise the possibility of systemic toxicity, as discussed earlier.

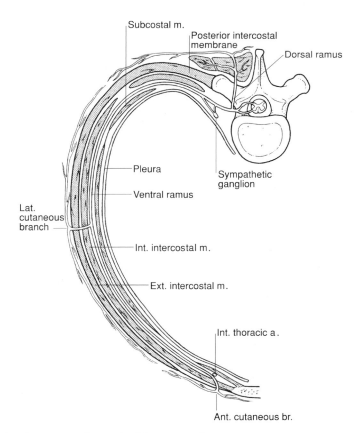

Fig. 2.8 Anatomy of a typical intercostal nerve. a. = artery; m. = muscle.

Intercostal nerve block

Indications

An intercostal nerve block is a useful technique for providing unilateral segmental analgesia of the abdomen and thorax, either post-operatively for unilateral incisions such as cholecystectomy or for fractured ribs.

Anatomy

The intercostal nerves, formed from the anterior primary rami of the corresponding thoracic nerves, run with the intercostal vessels beneath their respective ribs. This neurovascular bundle lies in the subcostal groove, deep to the intercostal muscles, on the pleura posteriorly and the subcostal muscle anterolaterally (Fig. 2.8). Local anaesthetic injected around one nerve may thus spread to affect the adjacent intercostal spaces (Fig. 2.9).

Technique

Site the injection proximal to the posterior axillary line (to ensure block of the lateral cutaneous branch). Place the patient in the sitting

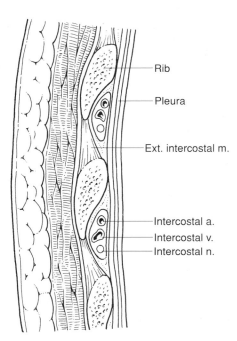

— Rib

— Pleura

— Ext. intercostal m.

— Intercostal a.
— Intercostal v.
— Intercostal n.

Fig. 2.9 Schematic cross-section through two intercostal spaces at the angle of the rib.

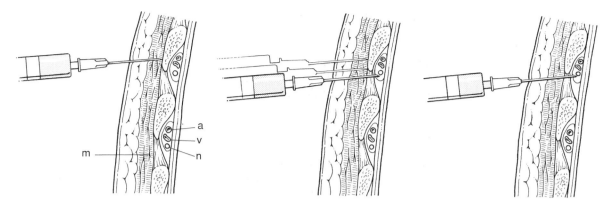

Fig. 2.10   Intercostal nerve block. a. = artery; v. = vein; m. = muscle; n. = nerve.

position with the shoulders abducted and the arms forward, leaning over two or three pillows. Locate the posterior angle of the ribs and at this point introduce a 25 gauge short-bevel needle at right angles to the skin until it comes into contact with the lower half of the rib. At this point, inject a small amount of local anaesthetic on to the periosteum and 'walk' the needle off the bone inferiorly. Identify the inferior edge of the rib and ask the patient to hold his/her breath. Insert the needle a further 2 mm, through the posterior intercostal membrane but not the pleura (Fig. 2.10).

Aspiration should be performed to exclude intravascular or pleural placement and 3–5 ml of local anaesthetic should be injected slowly. Bupivacaine 0.25% with 1:200 000 adrenaline is suitable but care should be exercised if many nerves are blocked or repeated injections are made, because of the rapid systemic absorption from this site with its attendant risk of toxicity. Prilocaine 0.5–1.0% with 1:200 000 adrenaline is a safer drug, but has a substantially shorter duration of action.

Bilateral blocks should be avoided because of the risk of pneumothorax, but several blocks may be performed on the same side.

> Ask the patient to breath very gently and hold his breath once the needle is in position to decrease the risk of pneumothorax.

Complications

The most common complication, pneumothorax (0.075–19%), can be avoided by careful technique. It is usually self-limiting and seldom requires drainage. If coughing is provoked the needle should be withdrawn, since it may be due to pleural irritation. If there is any suggestion of pneumothorax a chest X-ray must be examined as soon as possible.

Local anaesthetic toxicity may occur if multiple injections are made, since systemic absorption is rapid from this highly vascular area.

Haemorrhage, although a risk, is seldom a problem; occasionally surgical intervention is required to ligate a bleeding intercostal artery.

Hypotension has been reported due to posterior spread of local anaesthetic to the sympathetic chain.

INTRAVENOUS SEDATION

Definition

Sedation is a state of depressed consciousness in which verbal contact is maintained with the patient. It is usually characterized by anxiolysis, amnesia and hypnosis.

General considerations

Pharmacological sedation may be administered by several routes but the intravenous method is usually preferred and will be discussed below, with brief mention of the circumstances under which alternative routes may be more appropriate.

The drugs commonly used to produce sedation do not provide analgesia; sedation should never be considered an alternative to adequate analgesia. Used in conjunction with local or regional analgesia it enhances operating conditions in those patients in whom a general anaesthetic is not considered appropriate.

All sedative drugs produce CNS depression to a greater or lesser extent and their use must therefore be monitored carefully by an appropriately trained individual not directly involved in the procedure. Overdosage is associated with respiratory depression and the loss of airway maintenance and protective reflexes. Vigilance is particularly important where other depressant drugs (such as narcotic analgesics) have been administered, the effects of which may be additive or synergistic and may result in profound respiratory depression.

The administration of supplementary oxygen will maintain oxygen saturation in the presence of minor hypoventilation but is no substitute for care and caution in the use of sedation. As a general rule, preset doses of a drug should be avoided: intravenous administration should be slowly titrated against the patient's response until the desired level of sedation has been achieved.

Particular care should be exercised in the management of the elderly and sick, since the combination of a greatly enhanced sensitivity to depressant drugs and their slow circulation times make them particularly susceptible to overdose.

Choice of agent for sedation

Benzodiazepines

These are the most suitable and commonly used agents for intravenous sedation. They act centrally to enhance the release of GABA (gamma-aminobutyric acid), an inhibitory neurotransmitter causing presynaptic inhibition in many areas of the brain, particularly in the limbic and reticular activating systems.

Used correctly they are safe drugs but in excess they may cause profound respiratory depression and result in airway obstruction sufficient to cause hypoxia and respiratory arrest.

There is a specific antagonist available – flumazenil – and this should be at hand whenever benzodiazepines are used for intravenous sedation. Flumazenil should be administered in a dose of 0.5–1.0 mg; it acts rapidly and its effects persist for 2–3 hours.

Diazepam   This is a highly lipid-soluble drug, which is presented in an aqueous solution (with propylene glycol, which causes pain on injection) or in a lipid emulsion in water, which is much less irritant. The dose required by healthy adults is 0.15–0.2 mg/kg, but titration of the dose against the clinical response is more reliable. Diazepam acts within 5 minutes (therefore titration should be performed slowly) and has a variable duration of action of around 4–6 hours.

It may be given orally 30–60 minutes prior to surgery, in doses of 10–15 mg, but the response is much more variable.

Midazolam   This has now largely replaced diazepam for use in intravenous sedation, because of its similar onset time but shorter duration of action of around 30–60 minutes. It is both lipid- and water-soluble and is available in solutions of 2 mg/ml or 5 mg/ml, the former being easier to titrate against response in small, controlled doses. It is not irritant on injection.

The usual dose required for sedation is in the range 0.05–0.1 mg/kg, although elderly patients may require as little as 1 mg to produce quite marked sedation. It produces good anterograde, but not retrograde, amnesia, with anxiolysis and drowsiness. In larger doses it will cause marked respiratory depression and may induce general anaesthesia.

Temazepam   This short-acting benzodiazepine is available orally and, while it is commonly used as a premedicant before general anaesthesia, it is also suitable for use as a sedative in combination with analgesia or alone.

It is given as a tablet 1 hour prior to surgery, in a dose of 0.2–0.5 mg/kg, and will produce good quality sedation and anxiolysis. A syrup preparation is available for paediatric use.

> The duration of action of flumazenil is shorter than that of many benzodiazepines and there is therefore a risk of delayed recurrence of respiratory depression. Patients who have received flumazenil should be observed for a period exceeding the duration of effect of the benzodiazepine originally administered.

Lorazepam This long-acting benzodiazepine is useful as a premedicant in particularly anxious patients because of its marked anxiolysis and amnesia but is seldom used specifically for its sedative properties during surgical procedures. As a premedicant it is used in doses of 1–5 mg orally. It has benefits when used as a nocturnal sedative in very anxious patients the night before surgery.

Phenothiazines

These agents have been superseded by the benzodiazepines for sedation during surgery. They are used in adults for their antiemetic properties (prochlorperazine 12.5 mg) but are still occasionally used as sedative premedicants in children (promethazine, trimeprazine). They have numerous side-effects, including acute dystonias, extrapyramidal movements, anticholinergic symptoms and alpha-blockade-mediated hypotension, and these have restricted their use.

POSTOPERATIVE ANALGESIA

General principles

Adequate postoperative analgesia has direct benefits beyond the simply humanitarian. Respiratory function is improved, sputum clearance is facilitated and the adverse cardiovascular effects associated with pain, peripheral vasoconstriction, tachycardia and hypertension are minimized.

Regular administration may result in a decrease in total analgesic requirements compared with an 'as required' regime.

The simultaneous use of drugs with different mechanisms of action results in an improvement in the quality of analgesia and reduces opiate requirements.

Simple analgesics

Paracetamol is a central prostaglandin inhibitor with analgesic and antipyretic actions that readily crosses the blood–brain barrier. There is a risk of acute hepatocellular damage and fulminant hepatic failure following the administration of large doses, particularly in patients taking alcohol or barbiturates.

Non-steroidal anti-inflammatory drugs (NSAIDs)

Mechanism of action

This large group of drugs includes the substituted acids (aspirin, indomethacin), the propionic acid derivatives (ibuprofen,

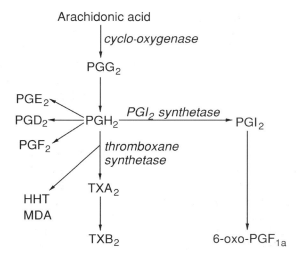

Fig. 2.11 Prostaglandin synthetic pathway, showing site of action of NSAIDs.

naproxen, ketoprofen) and the pyrazolones (phenylbutazone, oxyphenbutazone). Their common mode of action is to inhibit cyclo-oxygenase, thus decreasing peripheral prostaglandin production and consequently reducing inflammatory mediators, leading to their anti-pyretic, anti-inflammatory and analgesic actions (Fig. 2.11). The nature and sites of cyclo-oxygenase inhibition differ between agents, accounting for the variation seen in the predominant actions of different drugs.

Toxicity

Although they are very useful drugs when used correctly, the NSAIDs do have a number of potential side-effects. They may precipitate renal failure in patients with compromised renal function, by inhibition of the protective effect of renal prostaglandins. They may provoke bronchospasm in susceptible individuals. There is a significant risk of peptic ulceration during long-term use of NSAIDs in high doses, associated with haemorrhage and significant morbidity. By preferential inhibition of cyclo-oxygenase in vascular endothelium, the NSAIDs in low dose inhibit the formation of vascular thromboxane $A_{#2}$ (platelet-aggregating), with relatively little effect on platelet prostacyclin production. The overall effect is to reduce platelet aggregation and to decrease platelet function, with the risk of enhanced bleeding in some situations. When administered in large doses, inhibition of prostacyclin production obviates this effect.

Contraindications

Non-steroidals should be avoided in anyone with a history of bronchospasm or allergy following previous exposure. They should be avoided in patients with a history of active peptic ulceration and only used with care, for short periods, in anyone with a previous history of dyspeptic symptoms. They are contraindicated in patients with existing renal impairment, and great care should be taken in the elderly unless renal function has been checked. Aspirin must not be given to children because of the risk of Reye's syndrome.

Indications

Non-steroidal drugs are excellent analgesics, particularly for non-visceral soft-tissue and bone pain. They are most effective when given regularly in order to establish a background level of analgesia, and will considerably reduce the requirement for postoperative opiates when used in this fashion. They may be given orally, rectally and, in the case of ketorolac, intramuscularly.

They are of great value in day-case surgery and for many minor operations may be the only analgesia required.

Choice of drug

There are dozens of non-steroidals available, often differing very slightly in their side-effect profile. As a general rule, given in adequate dose, they all have roughly the same analgesic potential. A few commonly used and well-tested drugs are described below, and it is suggested that, in view of their similarity, the reader endeavours to become familiar with one or two examples.

- **Ibuprofen**:
  - orally 100–200 mg, three or four times a day, up to 1.2–1.8 g daily if required;
- **Naproxen**:
  - orally 250 mg every 6–8 hours;
  - rectally 500 mg suppositories 12–24-hourly;
- **Diclofenac**:
  - orally 75–150 mg daily in divided doses;
  - rectally 100 mg suppositories 18–24-hourly;
  - maximum dose 150 mg/24 h;
  - avoid i.m. injection because of risk of sterile abscess formation;
- **Ketorolac**:
  - a relatively new drug, which seems to have greater potency than other NSAIDs but is not antipyretic and has minimal anti-inflammatory effect;

- orally 10 mg every 6 hours;
- by i.m. injection 10 mg up to 4–6-hourly;
- maximum dose 60 mg/24 h;
- onset of analgesia 30 minutes after i.v./i.m., peak effect 1–2 hours;
- no more than 2 days treatment by either route.

Narcotic analgesics

Indications

Drugs synthesized from and related to opium have been used for their analgesic properties for many centuries. Opium (Greek = 'juice') is obtained from the latex of poppy heads and contains morphine and other alkaloids such as papaverine, thebaine, codeine and narcotine. The older opioids, such as morphine and papaveretum, are simply purified extract of opium, but many of the newer drugs are synthetic or semi-synthetic and have different time courses of action, although their properties are broadly speaking the same. Morphine is the standard against which all the other agents are compared.

Properties of morphine

CNS   There is analgesia to all forms of pain, but especially dull visceral pain, and this is associated with euphoria, drowsiness and a feeling of well-being. As larger doses are given there is progression to sedation, sleep and ultimately deep unconsciousness.

Respiratory   There is dose-dependent depression of ventilation (largely due to a reduction in tidal volume) and suppression of cough and airway reflexes.

Gastrointestinal   Nausea and vomiting are common, as a result of stimulation of the chemoreceptor trigger zone. There is decreased peristalsis, slowed gastric emptying and constipation. There is increased non-peristaltic smooth muscle tone, which may cause spasm of the ureters, fallopian tubes and bowel sphincters.

Endocrine   There is stimulation of the adrenal medulla, with increased catecholamine levels, and increased release of ADH from the posterior pituitary.

Addiction   This is both physical and psychological addiction, which may lead to an acute withdrawal reaction 8–12 hours after the last dose.

Other features   There is miosis from central stimulation, there may be bradycardia and hypotension, although unpredictable, and there may be histamine release with bronchospasm, erythema and hypotension. Tolerance develops to the opiates quite quickly with continued use and progressively larger doses are needed to achieve the same pharmacological effect.

Precautions

The most common problems are due to respiratory depression and narcotics should be used cautiously, if at all, in patients with respiratory compromise.

All the effects of the opiates are antagonized by **naloxone**, which should be administered i.v. in 100 µg increments until a response is achieved. It must be remembered that naloxone may have a shorter duration of action than the opiate it reverses and that there is therefore the potential for respiratory depression to recur.

Choice of drug

The following are suitable for the relief of postoperative pain. They should routinely be given with an antiemetic in the postoperative setting.

- **Morphine** remains the standard against which all others are judged. **Dose:** for acute pain 0.1–0.25 mg/kg i.m. or s.c. up to 4-hourly; alternatively, 0.035 mg/kg i.v. given slowly with careful observation and, if necessary, repeated. The full effect is achieved after 10–15 minutes i.v., or 15–30 minutes i.m. or s.c.
- **Diamorphine** has twice the potency of morphine, a more rapid onset of action and is more likely to produce euphoria and addiction; it is used for severe pain associated with cancer and myocardial infarction. **Dose:** 0.07–0.2 mg/kg i.m. or 0.03–0.07 mg/kg i.v., slowly.
- **Pethidine** is one-tenth as potent as morphine and is shorter-acting, with a more rapid onset of action. Because of its lack of histamine release it is safer than morphine for asthmatic or atopic individuals. **Dose:** 1–2 mg/kg every 3–4 hours i.m. or s.c.
- **Buprenorphine** has both agonist and antagonist actions at opiate receptors and there is therefore a ceiling to its clinical effect; given sublingually it is rapid-acting but commonly causes nausea and dysphoria; because of its agonist/antagonist actions it should not be used in conjunction with other opiates, when it may precipitate an acute withdrawal reaction. **Dose:** 200–400 µg sublingually every 8 hours.

- **Codeine phosphate** is a weaker opiate for mild to moderate pain, which may be given by mouth or intramuscular injection; it causes less sedation and respiratory depression and is therefore popular for use in head-injured patients. **Dose**: 30–60 mg orally or i.m. every 4 hours.

Patient-controlled analgesia (PCA)

Pain is a subjective experience and there are large variations in postoperative analgesic requirements, both between patients and with time in an individual. Intermittent injections, even given regularly, often result in considerable variation in the quality of analgesia provided. The development of patient-controlled analgesia, by giving control back to the patient, has to a large extent overcome this problem by allowing patients to titrate the administration of narcotics to their own needs. Pain control is improved while overall opiate requirements are decreased. The patient must be cooperative and should understand and be physically capable of operating the equipment.

The pump   Most pumps allow the operator to programme the size of the bolus dose to be given, the interval between administration of successive doses (the lockout duration), the maximum dose to be administered in a 4-hour period and the rate of background infusion (if required).

The patient control system   This consists of a handset or wristwatch button which, when depressed, initiates the administration of the predetermined bolus dose.

Drugs used   Morphine, papaveretum, diamorphine and pethidine are all suitable. Morphine at a concentration of 1 mg/ml is the accepted standard, but this may be increased to 2 mg/ml or more in patients with high narcotic requirements.

Safety   Regular observations must be performed on any patient receiving narcotics, and these should include respiratory rate and sedation scoring as well as the usual postoperative observations. The nursing staff supervising the use of PCA must be trained in the operation of the equipment and familiar with its limitations.

INSERTION OF CENTRAL VENOUS LINES

Percutaneous internal jugular and subclavian vein cannulation in inexperienced hands is associated with local haematoma, pneumothorax, haemothorax, air and catheter embolus, arterial puncture and sepsis. However, the insertion of a central venous cannula is now commonplace and, performed with care, should be within the sphere of competence of all surgical trainees. There are several approaches to cannulation of a central vein, but the two described are well established, with clear landmarks.

Indications

- To permit the measurement of central venous pressure (CVP). Central venous pressure measurement facilitates the accurate assessment of the volume status of a patient, particularly where clinical signs may be inaccurate. It is particularly useful in patients with poorly functioning hearts, in those subject to large, rapid or covert fluid losses, during rapid fluid administration and in those patients whose ability to regulate their own fluid balance is impaired.
- To permit the administration into a central vein of drugs that are potentially harmful if administered peripherally (e.g. catecholamines, potassium or parenteral nutrition).

Contraindications

There are no absolute contraindications to CVP line placement.

Exercise great care in patients with a bleeding diathesis or clotting abnormality, when experienced help should be sought.

Local sepsis precludes a site from cannulation.

In severe respiratory disease, particularly bullous emphysema, the lower risk of pneumothorax should encourage the use of the internal jugular rather than the subclavian approach.

Technique

Equipment CVP lines may be inserted by threading the catheter through or over a needle, or by the use of a guide wire. This latter, the Seldinger technique, is the most frequently employed and is probably the easiest for the occasional user. It involves the introduction of a needle connected to a syringe into the chosen vessel. Once the lumen has been identified, the syringe is removed, taking care not to displace the needle, and a flexible guide wire is passed into the vein. The needle can then be removed, leaving an intravenous guide wire over which dilators and the catheter can be introduced safely. The guide wire is finally removed.

Asepsis A strict aseptic technique is essential.

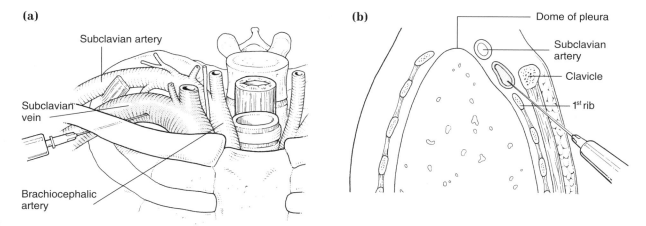

Fig. 2.12 Anatomy of the infraclavicular approach to the subclavian vein. **(a)** Anterior. **(b)** Sagittal.

Subclavian vein cannulation

General

The subclavian vein is best cannulated by the infraclavicular approach, particularly if prolonged use is anticipated, since subcutaneous tunnelling is facilitated. While it is more comfortable for the patient it is best avoided in patients with emphysema, marked respiratory compromise or those being positive-pressure ventilated, because of the risk of pneumothorax.

Technique

Place the patient supine in a 20° head-down tilt, arms at his/her sides, and turn the head away from the side to be punctured. Mark the medial and lateral ends of the clavicle, the rostral end of the sternum and the heads of sternocleidomastoid. Identify the junction of the middle and medial thirds of the clavicle through the skin and, if the patient is conscious, infiltrate 5–10 ml of local anaesthetic through the skin, down on to the periosteum of the clavicle and first rib. Insert a needle at this point (Fig. 2.12) just deep to the clavicle, over the first rib, and direct it slightly cephalad towards the sternal notch.

Continually aspirate the syringe plunger as the needle is advanced, and a positive flashback of blood indicates entry into the subclavian vein, usually at a depth of less than 5 cm. Insert the catheter using the Seldinger technique, as described above.

Once secured in position, arrange a chest X-ray to ensure that the tip of the line lies in the superior vena cava and to exclude a pneumothorax.

> Puncture is facilitated by placing a sandbag or litre bag of i.v. fluid longitudinally beneath the upper thoracic vertebrae in order to displace the shoulders dorsally.

Complications

There may be a pneumothorax requiring pleural drainage. The subclavian artery may be punctured with significant haemorrhage, and there may be local haematoma formation.

Internal jugular vein cannulation

General

Because the incidence of complications is low, even when performed by the relatively inexperienced operator, the internal jugular vein route is to be preferred in most situations where short-term central venous access is required. Catheterization of the right side is preferred since the right internal jugular and brachiocephalic veins and the superior vena cava lie in an almost straight line.

The internal jugular vein runs immediately lateral to the carotid artery behind the sternocleidomastoid muscle and may be cannulated at a point midway between the mastoid process and the

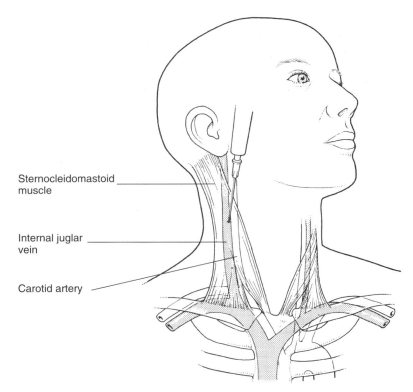

Fig. 2.13   Cannulation of the internal jugular vein.

sternal notch. If the carotid pulse is palpated at this point the internal jugular vein lies just lateral to it (Fig. 2.13).

Technique

Place the patient supine in 20° of Trendelenburg. Gently extend the neck by placing a pillow behind the shoulders and turn the head half away from the side to be used. Identify the carotid artery at the midpoint of sternocleidomastoid and inject a small volume of local anaesthetic subcutaneously. Introduce a needle connected to a syringe at an angle of 30° to the skin, immediately lateral to the carotid pulse, and direct it caudally and laterally towards the ipsilateral nipple.

The internal jugular vein should be entered at a depth of 3–4 cm. If it is not identified then direct the needle more laterally. Failure to cannulate the internal jugular vein often results from the needle being introduced too laterally in an attempt to avoid carotid artery puncture.

Complications

Internal jugular cannulation is not infrequently associated with puncture of the internal carotid artery and complicated by haemorrhage; the approach should be avoided in the presence of carotid artery disease and used with caution in the presence of a coagulopathy. If too low an approach is made, pneumothorax is still a possibility and a chest X-ray should be taken to confirm correct placement.

Identification of the site of the internal jugular vein with a 23 gauge needle introduced exactly as above, before introduction of the large Seldinger needle, will minimize the consequences of inadvertent carotid puncture.

Medical problems in the surgical patient

3

Brian A. Leatherdale

This chapter will deal with the common medical problems encountered by a junior doctor on the general surgical wards. These will be considered in two sections, acute medical problems developing postoperatively and management of existing common medical problems perioperatively.

ACUTE MEDICAL PROBLEMS

When patients collapse following surgical treatment you must exclude possible complications of the surgical procedure, but, with the increasing number of elderly patients with pre-existing medical problems requiring surgical treatment, medical causes of collapse are increasing in importance. Cases of collapse not directly due to the surgical procedure include the following.

Acute coronary thrombosis

This can occur at any stage during a patient's admission and may affect patients not previously known to be suffering from ischaemic heart disease. Patients with established coronary artery disease are at greater risk and require careful preoperative assessment and expert anaesthesia.

The patient will typically complain of central chest pain of a 'crushing' nature, which radiates into the upper arms, back or front of the neck. Pain localized just to the precordium is very unlikely to be cardiac. In patients with coronary thrombosis the presence of nausea and sweating may be helpful in distinguishing from anginal attacks. Take a careful history to separate upper abdominal pain following abdominal surgery from chest pain.

The outcome of coronary thrombosis will depend on the extent of the lesion and whether dysrhythmias develop. The most critical period is immediately following the thrombosis and up to 4–6 hours later, so a rapid diagnosis is necessary. If the lesion is very extensive, the patient's cardiac output will fall rapidly, with a tachycardia and hypotension, peripheral vasoconstriction and sweating (cardiogenic shock). This may also result from a dysrhythmia. Examine the patient, looking for a third heart sound or raised JVP and signs of left ventricular failure. Perform an ECG, which will confirm the diagnosis in most cases and will establish the heart rhythm. Look carefully at the ECG for signs of acute injury, i.e. raised ST segments in the inferior leads II, III and AVF and/or anterior leads V1–V6 (Fig. 3.1). When the diagnosis is confirmed, move the patient to a bed with a cardiac monitor, preferably in a coronary care unit, for further management.

Acute massive pulmonary embolus

Always consider acute massive pulmonary embolus in patients who collapse after surgical treatment. The usual source of the embolus is in the deep veins of the legs, with extension above the knee or in the pelvic veins. Pulmonary embolus more commonly follows operations for neoplasms and gynaecological and orthopaedic procedures (particularly hip replacement). Surgery predisposes to venous thrombosis because of Virchow's triad of abnormalities, which frequently occur postoperatively:

- damage to the wall of the vein;
- stasis of blood within the vessel;
- increased blood coagulability.

The problem frequently occurs between 5 and 10 days postoperatively in a 'convalescent' patient.

The patient characteristically complains of acute shortness of breath with a varying degree of chest discomfort. On examination there is a rapid heart rate, hypotension and peripheral vasoconstriction with sweating and central cyanosis. The venous pressure will be elevated, there may be a loud second heart sound and a parasternal lift indicating right ventricular strain. Look for signs of deep venous thrombosis, i.e. oedema, calf tenderness and tenderness over the femoral vein. These signs, however, can be misleading. There may be slight pyrexia. Obtain an ECG, although this is rarely very helpful diagnostically; it may reveal signs of right heart strain with an S wave in lead I and Q wave with inverted T in lead III (S1, Q3, T3). Chest X-ray is rarely helpful but may reveal pulmonary oligaemia. The diagnosis is, however, often one of exclusion, so that chest X-ray and ECG will exclude other causes of collapse (e.g. coronary thrombosis, collapsed lobe, chest infection). When the index of suspicion is high, intravenous heparin and 35% oxygen should be given without delay.

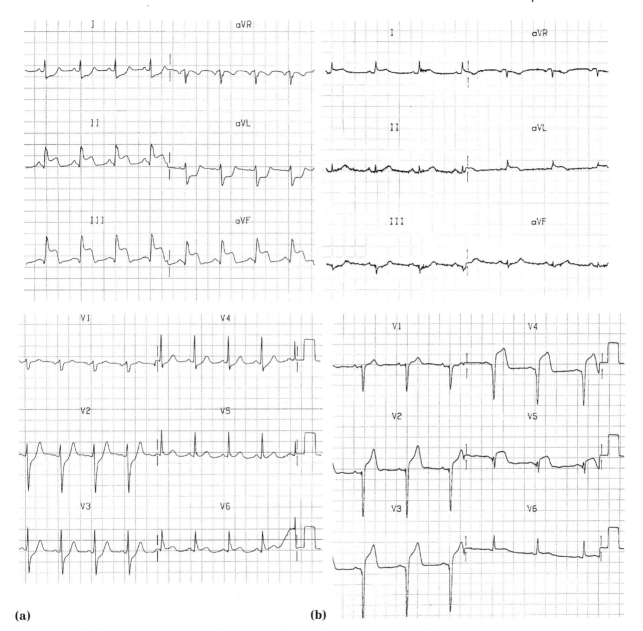

(a)   (b)

Fig. 3.1   (a) The typical changes of an inferior myocardial infarction, with raised ST segments in leads 2, 3 and AVF. **(b)** The classical changes of an anterior myocardial infarction, with ST segment elevation in leads V2–V6 and also in AVL.

The outcome of acute pulmonary embolus depends on the size of the clot and, if the patient survives for the initial 2–3 hours, the outlook is good. Continue oxygen and heparin therapy and monitor the patient for cardiac dysrhythmias. The use of streptokinase is controversial but consider it if the patient's condition fails to improve despite adequate heparinization. Surgical intervention should be reserved for patients who fail to improve with streptokinase, as the mortality from emergency embolectomy is extremely high. Fortunately, patients who do not immediately perish usually recover completely. Intravenous heparin should be continued for 7 days after the event; anticoagulate the patient with warfarin for at least a further 6 months.

Septicaemia

This is more common after abdominal operations, particularly emergency procedures for acute perforation of a viscus, and in immunocompromised patients. It can also occur after trauma, e.g. stab wounds. With improved surgical techniques and the use of prophylactic antibiotics its incidence is falling. On examination the septicaemic patient is often confused and disorientated with no focal neurological signs. The patient is frequently pyrexial and hypotensive with a rapid heart rate but no signs of heart failure. The hypotension is associated with peripheral vasodilatation and the cardiac output is increased, so that the peripheries are warm and well perfused rather than cold and vasoconstricted as is the case in coronary thrombosis or pulmonary embolus. The patient will usually have a normal chest X-ray (unless a chest infection is the cause); the ECG will be normal and the patient is usually breathless. Take blood cultures and urine and sputum for culture where appropriate. Blood count will usually show a polymorphonuclear leucocytosis; check the platelets, clotting screen and fibrin degradation products to exclude disseminated intravascular coagulation (DIC). Obtain plasma creatinine, urea and electrolytes to have a baseline.

Resuscitate the patient with intravenous fluids and possibly plasma expanders and/or blood, and give intravenous antibiotics. The choice of antibiotics will depend on the 'best guess' of the probable organism responsible; do not delay treatment until cultures are available. In many cases the cause is the Gram-negative bacillus *Escherichia coli*, so choose a broad-spectrum antibiotic active against *E. coli*. Gentamicin and the cephalosporins are normally used. In elderly patients monitor venous pressure with a central venous line.

Acute collapse of a lung or lobe of lung

This is an unusual cause of postoperative collapse except in patients recovering from thoracic surgical procedures. It can, however, occur in patients after upper abdominal procedures and is more common in smokers and patients with obstructive airways disease in whom sputum retention occurs. The patient may have been complaining of a productive cough for some days and may then develop sudden onset of acute shortness of breath. In young patients, with relatively normal lung function perioperatively, lobar collapse may be very well tolerated but in older patients with compromised lung function collapse may cause severe hypoxia. On examination the patient will be dyspnoeic with a tachycardia and normal blood pressure, cyanosis may be present and the trachea will be deviated to the side of the lesion if the upper lobes are involved. In collapse of the left lower lobe the apex beat will be displaced laterally. There will be no signs of heart failure. A chest X-ray will reveal the extent of the collapse but left lower lobe collapse may be missed unless specifically looked for, as the collapsed lower lobe is hidden by the heart shadow which is then displaced laterally with some elevation of the left hemidiaphragm. Treat this condition with antibiotics and vigorous physiotherapy. This usually leads to expansion of the lobe but bronchoscopy may very occasionally be required to remove tenacious plugs of sputum. When you give oxygen to patients with chronic obstructive airways disease, always monitor blood gases carefully.

Tension pneumothorax

This is a very rare diagnosis, which must be considered in patients who collapse postoperatively with dyspnoea. It is more common in young men. On examination, the patient is increasingly dyspnoeic with rapid pulse and normal/raised blood pressure; there are no signs of heart failure. The trachea is deviated away from the side of the lesion; percussion note is normal but breath sounds are diminished on the affected side (this can, however, be very difficult to assess in the severely dyspnoeic patient). For signs of subcutaneous emphysema, which is often evident, carefully palpate the supraclavicular fossae. Request a very urgent chest X-ray and remove air urgently from the affected side. If the patient is *in extremis* and the diagnosis is clinically very likely, decompress the lung using a 50 ml syringe, with a wide-bore needle attached and the plunger removed. Insert the needle into the midclavicular line in the appropriate second intercostal space.

PERIOPERATIVE MANAGEMENT OF COMMON MEDICAL PROBLEMS

Postoperative chest pain

A careful history is of enormous value. The nature of the chest pain usually gives a clue to the diagnosis and the age of the patient should be taken into account in assessing the likely causes. The main differential diagnoses to be considered are pain from ischaemic heart disease and pain due to pulmonary emboli. The pain of myocardial ischaemia is usually felt retrosternally, is never described as pleu-

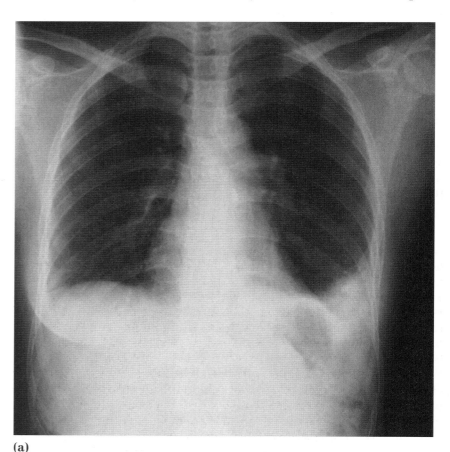

(a)

Fig. 3.2 **(a)** Chest X-ray and **(b)** Ventilation (*V*.) and perfusion (*Q*.) scans of a patient with multiple pulmonary emboli. The chest X-ray is normal apart from a possible small area of linear atelectasis at the left base. The posterior (P) and right posterior oblique (RPO) *V./Q*. scans show typical mismatched ventilated but non-perfused segments of lung.

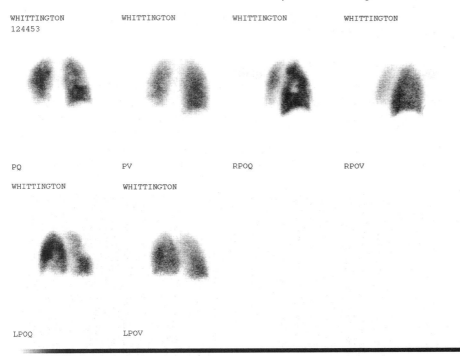

WHITTINGTON
124453

WHITTINGTON

WHITTINGTON

WHITTINGTON

PQ

PV

RPOQ

RPOV

WHITTINGTON

WHITTINGTON

LPOQ

LPOV

(b)

Fig. 3.2 *Continued*

ritic, frequently spreads to the neck, upper arms or back and is described as crushing or tight in nature. It tends to affect middle-aged men, who may have a previous history of exercise-induced angina. Distinguish it from oesophagitis, which also causes retrosternal discomfort, is more commonly described as burning and rarely radiates to the arms and neck. Oesophagitis is often exacerbated by eating and is usually relieved by antacids. Pulmonary embolus tends to occur 4–5 days after operation and can cause sudden collapse. Multiple small pulmonary emboli classically cause pleuritic chest pains associated with dyspnoea and haemoptysis. In such cases you may be able to detect a pleural rub over the site of the pain; examine the legs for evidence of deep venous thrombosis, which may need to be confirmed with a duplex Doppler examination or venogram. Patients at risk are typically obese and may have varicose veins.

Always request a chest X-ray and ECG to evaluate patients complaining of postoperative chest pain. The ECG may show evidence of a coronary thrombosis or changes suggestive of ischaemia, but may be perfectly normal in angina. In cases of multiple small pulmonary emboli the chest X-ray may reveal areas of linear atelectasis or peripheral 'wedge-shaped' shadows, but is frequently normal. When you suspect pulmonary embolism, request a ventilation–perfusion scan (Fig. 3.2).

Unless the pulmonary embolus is large the ECG will show no change. Small pulmonary emboli may precede a massive embolus and such patients should receive treatment with intravenous heparin. Subsequently, warfarin is usually given for at least 6 weeks after diagnosis.

Other causes of chest pain include pneumonia, trauma to the chest wall during surgery, pericarditis, oesophagitis and 'scoline' pains. These can usually be distinguished from angina or pulmonary emboli by a careful history, examination, chest X-ray and ECG.

Diabetes mellitus

This is often a cause of anxiety for trainee surgeons because of the worry that patients are not able to eat their normal diet perioperatively. With careful monitoring and treatment, problems can be avoided and the diabetes can be kept under good control during even the most extensive surgery. The important goals should be to avoid hypoglycaemia, particularly under anaesthesia, and to prevent hyperglycaemia (blood glucose persistently over 10 mmol/l) so that recovery and wound healing are not impaired. Surgical procedures cause release of 'stress' hormones (cortisol, growth hormone and catecholamines) which antagonize the actions of insulin and in normal people this leads to increased insulin secretion. In insulin-dependent patients (IDDs) insulin administration will therefore frequently need to be increased temporarily perioperatively, and non-insulin-dependent (NIDDs) patients may require treatment with insulin perioperatively. It is convenient to consider patients under three categories.

Diet-controlled patients

Such patients will usually tolerate minor surgery without any special precautions but may require insulin during major surgical procedures. Send a sample for fasting laboratory blood glucose on the day of operation and after recovery from anaesthesia. Finger-prick blood samples should be measured every 6 hours using reagent strips until the patient is stable.

Tablet treated patients

Patients treated with diet and tablets normally tolerate minor surgery without incident but will normally require insulin peri-operatively during major surgery. They will usually be able to return to their preoperative regimen before discharge from hospital. Monitor these patients perioperatively as for diet-controlled patients. Stop long-acting sulphonylureas the evening before surgery and stop short-acting sulphonylureas on the operative day. Biguanides should also be stopped perioperatively. Start an insulin infusion in NIDD patients if blood glucose levels are above 10 mmol/l and maintain the infusion until the patient is stable (see below).

Patients on insulin

Such patients are best put first on the list.

For minor procedures lasting less than one hour   The patient who is on a twice-daily regimen with a longer-acting insulin given the previous evening can often have the morning insulin omitted and have a short-acting insulin before lunch. Give such patients their usual evening insulin.

In most other situations use a continuous insulin infusion   The most convenient method of giving insulin is *via* a syringe pump. Draw up 50 units of insulin and 50 ml of normal saline into a 50 ml syringe so that each millilitre contains one unit of insulin. Use 5% dextrose or 4% dextrose with 0.18% normal saline to maintain the blood glucose. Infuse insulin at 1–2 units per hour and adjust the rate to maintain blood glucose levels between 5 and 10 mmol/l. Check finger-prick blood glucose levels hourly and then 2–4-hourly when stable, to assess insulin requirements. Frequent adjustment of the insulin infusion rate is usually unnecessary and merely produces wide fluctuations in blood glucose. Sliding scales (Table 3.1) based on frequent blood glucose measurements are popular and usually safe, but are not a substitute for regular reappraisal of the patient.

Many patients are adequately controlled on 1–2 units of insulin per

> Do not use a sliding scale that does not give insulin when blood glucose levels are normal, as this leads to hyperglycaemia and overadjustments are then made. This produces undesirable swings in blood glucose from high to low levels.

Table 3.1   A typical sliding scale for continuous i.v. insulin administration *via* an insulin infusion pump

Blood glucose (mmol/l)	Insulin dose (Units/h)	i.v. infusion
Less than 4	1	
4–11	2	5% dextrose with
11–17	4	added potassium
More than 17	6	

hour, which provides an adequate basal insulin level. A constant infusion of glucose is maintained to prevent hypoglycaemia. Some patients may, however, require insulin at 4–8 units per hour.

If a syringe pump is not available, insulin can be given *via* the ordinary infusion set. Some authorities advocate 10 units of insulin in 500 ml of 10% dextrose to which 10 mmol of potassium are added but this can produce undesirable hyperglycaemia. Use either 5 or 10 units of insulin in 500 ml of 5% dextrose with added K^+ (Table 3.1).

It should be possible, using these methods, to maintain blood glucose levels between 5 and 10 mmol throughout the perioperative period. Start the patient on his/her usual regimen as soon as s/he is eating again. It is best to give twice-daily intermediate-acting insulin to provide adequate basal insulin levels rather than frequent doses of rapid-acting insulins preprandially in the immediate postoperative period.

Total pancreatectomy

These patients are a special case, as the operation inevitably produces an insulin-dependent diabetes whatever the preoperative diabetic state of the patient. In addition, the loss of all pancreatic glucagon makes the patient prone to hypoglycaemia. For this reason, aim to keep the blood sugar above 10 mmol/l. Avoid hyperglycaemia (>15 mmol) by careful monitoring. Make sure that the patient is seen by a diabetic specialist before discharge from hospital, because after total pancreatectomy lifelong supervision will be required and the period of adjustment to an insulin regimen after discharge from hospital needs careful management.

The patient with chronic liver disease

The liver is involved in the production of most of the clotting factors and so the risk of postoperative bleeding may be increased. Such patients should all have coagulation studies preoperatively. In patients with obstructive jaundice, hypoprothrombinaemia usually results from inadequate absorption of vitamin K and this can be readily corrected by injection of 10 mg vitamin K intramuscularly preoperatively. Fresh frozen plasma will correct other abnormalities of coagulation in patients with hepatocellular dysfunction but help should be sought from a haematologist when difficulties arise.

Patients with chronic liver disease need to have their renal function and electrolytes monitored carefully perioperatively and care is necessary when normal saline is infused. Some patients may require albumin infusions. Patients who are jaundiced need careful attention to fluid balance. Dehydration must be avoided and careful administration of mannitol and a fluid load during operation may reduce the incidence of renal failure postoperatively.

Hepatic encephalopathy may be precipitated in susceptible patients perioperatively. If detected either pre- or postoperatively, treat it with lactulose and a low-protein diet. Patients most at risk are those known to have portocaval shunting.

The patient with renal disease

Patients with chronic renal failure suffer from an inability to concentrate the urine. Give careful attention to fluid balance and obtain daily electrolyte estimations. It is wise to commence an overnight infusion of fluid on the night before operation to avoid dehydration. Subsequently, replace all urinary losses with appropriate intravenous fluids. Measure urinary electrolytes to help assess these needs. It is of course important also to replace other fluid losses (e.g. vomit and aspirates). Nephrotic patients may need infusions of albumin perioperatively. The management of patients on dialysis is beyond the scope of this chapter. Always manage such patients in close collaboration with a nephrologist.

The patient with respiratory disease

Patients with chronic bronchitis and emphysema or asthma are at high risk of pulmonary complications postoperatively, particularly after upper abdominal operations. Preoperatively, advise such patients to stop smoking where appropriate. If their sputum is infected, give antibiotics. Pre- and postoperative physiotherapy has been shown to reduce morbidity; encourage the patients to mobilize as soon as clinically possible. Obtain blood gas analysis routinely preoperatively and when clinically indicated postoperatively. Peak flow rates are easily measured; monitor these regularly. Beta-agonists should be continued or started if appropriate, prescribe theophyllines if necessary. Prescribe antibiotics without delay to patients producing infected sputum.

The patient with established cardiac disease

Such patients are commonly encountered undergoing non-cardiac surgery. They fall into three main categories:

- patients with ischaemic heart disease;
- patients with chronic heart failure;
- patients with valvular heart disease.

Such patients need careful evaluation.

Patients with ischaemic heart disease

Patients with stable angina (i.e. patients who can walk up a flight of stairs without difficulties and who may be taking regular medication) do not seem to be at major risk from surgery. Continue their medication perioperatively and keep a close watch for signs of heart failure, which may signal a myocardial infarction. Patients with worse angina or who have had a recent myocardial infarction (within 6 months) have a very substantial risk of perioperative myocardial infarction and death and need very careful cardiac monitoring perioperatively. Consider myocardial revascularization procedures before elective non-cardiac surgery is performed in these patients.

Patients with chronic stable heart failure

These patients need careful attention perioperatively. Continue their medication and give it parenterally with dose adjustment where necessary. Particular care is necessary to avoid fluid overload and intravenous infusions should be planned to avoid excessive administration of saline.

Patients with heart valve lesions

These patients should have an echocardiogram, chest X-ray and ECG preoperatively. In most instances problems will not be encountered perioperatively if radiologically there is no cardiomegaly. Appropriate prophylaxis to avoid subacute bacterial endocarditis should be given.

Miscellaneous problems

Drugs and anaesthesia

Continue most current medications perioperatively and manage patients on steroids and diabetic patients as discussed above.

Table 3.2 Drugs that can cause problems during anaesthesia

Drug	Desirable drug-free interval prior to surgery
Monoamine oxidase inhibitors	2–3 weeks
Lithium carbonate	72 hours
Levodopa	Omit on day of surgery
Tricyclic antidepressants	72 hours
Contraceptive pill	1 month
Phenothiazines	72 hours

The drugs shown in Table 3.2 can cause problems during anaesthesia and for routine surgery should be stopped as indicated.

The patient with a bleeding disorder

The most important factor in identifying such patients is to take a careful history. A history of abnormal bleeding following minor trauma or dental extraction and patients who complain of easy bruising or who have hepatosplenomegaly on examination require investigations. Always ask for such a history. The investigations required are beyond the scope of this chapter: discuss such cases with a haematologist.

Patients who have taken steroids in the past

Patients may have taken steroids for polymyalgia rheumatica, asthma or a variety of rheumatic conditions and enquiry should always be made about use of such drugs. If patients have taken moderate doses of steroids (e.g. greater than 10 mg of prednisolone or equivalent) continuously for more than 2 months within the last 12 months, cover the perioperative period with 100 mg of hydrocortisone intramuscularly twice a day for 2–3 days.

Alcohol withdrawal syndrome

This may go unrecognized, particularly as alcoholics may conceal the true extent of their drinking habit. It should be suspected if a patient becomes confused 3–4 days postoperatively particularly if s/he appears agitated, sweaty, hypertensive and tremulous. Such patients may need treatment with intravenous heminevrin.

Hypertension

Patients with stable well-controlled hypertension can usually omit their drugs for a few days perioperatively and resume medication when stable again. In patients on diuretics, check the K^+ level preoperatively and correct any deficits prior to surgery.

Accident and emergency

Rodger A. Sleet and Mohammed A. Khan

4

The Accident and Emergency Department is responsible for the assessment and resuscitation of the severely injured and critically ill patient, as well as for the assessment and treatment of a wide variety of other injuries and acute illnesses. The basic surgical techniques required of the Accident Officer fall under the following headings:

- resuscitation;
- treatment of local infections such as paronychia and injuries to tissues;
- manipulation of common dislocations and fractures that can be managed under local or short-term general anaesthesia and after which the patient may be discharged home. (Fracture management is dealt with in Chapter 5.)

RESUSCITATION

The resuscitation of a severely injured patient in the UK follows standards established by the American College of Surgeons in the late 1970s and taught in the Advanced Trauma Life Support (ATLS) courses. The standards of management of severely injured patients are prioritized as shown in Table 4.1.

Primary assessment and resuscitation

Carry out assessment and resuscitation in the following priority:

- Airway (with cervical spine immobilized)
- Breathing
- Circulation.

Airway

The airway is at risk in the unconscious patient or in those with severe faciomaxillary trauma. In this group of patients there is a significant likelihood of associated cervical spine injury. Carry out any airway management manoeuvre with the neck immobilized in a

Table 4.1 Special steps in the resuscitation of a severely injured patients: observe this order of priorities

1. Primary assessment and resuscitation to identify and treat life-threatening conditions. Assessment and resuscitation take place simultaneously.
2. Limited neurological examination to identify neurological disability.
3. Expose the patient to allow a complete examination. At this stage obtain necessary X-rays of the cervical spine (lateral view), chest and pelvis, and take blood for arterial blood gas analysis and cross-matching.
4. Secondary assessment of potentially life-threatening conditions and management.
5. Carry out necessary definitive emergency treatment and complete patient records.
6. Transfer to the next stage of management.

semi-rigid collar supported with sandbags and with the head taped to the underlying examination trolley or preferably to a long spinal board. A patent airway is essential for survival and should have been obtained by the ambulance paramedic in the prehospital stage of management. To examine the airway lift the jaw forward to pull the tongue away from the oropharynx. This prevents obstruction by the tongue. Remove secretions with a gloved finger and wide-bore suction. To maintain the airway insert a suitably sized oropharyngeal tube. Depress the tongue with a spatula or laryngoscope blade and slide the airway over the tongue. Alternatively insert the airway with the concavity of the tube towards the soft palate and then rotate the airway over the tongue. Where an oropharyngeal airway fails to provide adequate protection and there is likelihood of vomiting, insert an endotracheal tube. Do not attempt this unless you have had specific training. The usual size for an adult man is 9.0 or 9.5, with one size smaller for an adult woman. Use an uncuffed tube for infants and small children. Give all injured patients high-concentration oxygen delivered *via* a tight-fitting facemask with reservoir (flow rates of 12–15 l/min).

Surgery to secure the airway

Severe facial injury may compromise the airway and oral intubation may be impossible. Under these circumstances a surgical approach is necessary. There are two methods available.

Needle cricothyroidotomy is the method of choice in children less than 12 years of age and can also be adopted as an emergency procedure in an adult. Remove the semi-rigid collar and have an assistant immobilize the neck manually.

Identify the cricothyroid membrane (Fig. 4.1).

Run a finger from the chin down the midline of the neck until the superior border of the thyroid cartilage is located. Identify the thyroid notch and pass your finger over the thyroid cartilage to locate the first space, which is the cricothyroid membrane. Clean the overlying skin with an antiseptic swab. Puncture the cricothyroid membrane using a 12 or 14 gauge catheter over a needle attached to a 5 ml syringe. Stabilize the trachea between your thumb and forefinger while you do this. Direct the needle at an angle of 45° through the membrane towards the chest, simultaneously aspirating the syringe. Confirm entry into the trachea by aspiration of air and then advance the cannula to its hub and detach the needle and syringe. Attach oxygen tubing to the catheter. If breathing is impaired ventilate the patient using a Y connection between the catheter and the oxygen tubing. Place a thumb over the open end of the

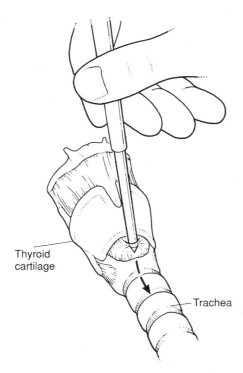

Thyroid cartilage

Trachea

Fig. 4.1 Needle cricothyroidotomy.

connector to close the system for 1 second and release for a further 4 seconds to allow for exhalation. Auscultate the chest to confirm adequate ventilation.

Needle cricothyroidotomy allows adequate oxygenation of the patient for approximately 30–40 min. Carbon dioxide accumulates towards the end of this time, which can compromise the management of patients with a head injury due to secondary swelling. Replace the cricothyroidotomy with endotracheal intubation or planned tracheostomy after 30 min.

Surgical cricothyroidotomy is the preferred management in the adult. Restrain the patient either on a long spinal board or manually with immobilization of the cervical spine and trunk. Remove the semi-rigid collar. Identify the cricothyroid membrane and immobilize the trachea between thumb and index finger as described above. In the conscious patient infiltrate the overlying skin with 2–3 ml of 1% lignocaine. Incise the skin overlying the cricothyroid membrane vertically and separate the edges with the thumb and forefinger; this provides haemostasis and exposes the cricothyroid membrane (Fig. 4.2).

Incise the membrane along its width. With the trachea fixed, dilate the incision with forceps or the handle of the scalpel to achieve an airway. Maintain and protect the airway by the insertion of a cuffed tracheostomy tube (4.0 or 4.5) and inflate the cuff with air. Use saline in the cuff if airborne evacuation is required. Secure the tube with

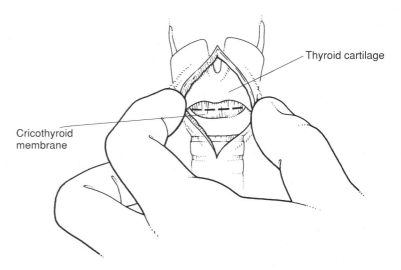

Thyroid cartilage

Cricothyroid membrane

Fig. 4.2   Incised skin revealing the cricothyroid membrane.

Table 4.2   Life-threatening chest injuries

- Tension pneumothorax
- Open pneumothorax
- Massive pneumothorax
- Flail chest with lung contusion
- Cardiac tamponade

tapes around the patient's neck. Connect an oxygen source to the tracheostomy tube and ventilate the patient either manually or mechanically. Close the wound with interrupted skin sutures and cover it with a sterile dressing. Finally, reapply the semi-rigid cervical collar.

> Take care not to incise the thyroid cartilage in this procedure.

Breathing

The immediately life-threatening chest injuries are shown in Table 4.2.

The resuscitation of patients with these injuries requires a clear airway, oxygenation, correction of hypovolaemic shock and, where indicated, wide-bore chest drain decompression. Fewer than 15% of these patients require formal thoracotomy.

Tension pneumothorax is a life-threatening emergency that you should suspect from the mechanism of injury and observed clinical signs. Do not wait for radiological examination of the patient, as this may delay life-saving intervention. Relieve the tension initially by the insertion of a 12 or 14 gauge cannula over a needle through the chest wall into the second intercostal space in the midclavicular line on the suspected side of the pneumothorax. Remove the needle. Audible escape of air confirms the diagnosis and relieves the underlying tension, allowing time for the necessary preparation for chest drain insertion.

The drain should be inserted into the fourth intercostal space on the affected side between the anterior and midaxillary line. Any incision lower than this level carries the risk of intra-abdominal injury, as the diaphragm rises to the level of the intercostal space during expiration.

Use the technique described in Chapter 1.

Flail chest requires immediate positive pressure ventilation to stabilize the fracture and to oxygenate both lungs. In the absence of facial injuries, ventilate using a mask until skilled assistance is available to intubate the patient.

> - Do not use a chest drain over a trocar as there is a risk of damaging the underlying lung and pulmonary vessels, or even of causing intra-abdominal injury
> - if there is a continuous air leak consider the possibility of a broncho-pleural fistula. Chest X-ray will show a pneumothorax; insert a second chest drain before making arrangements for formal thoracotomy.
> - if there is an open pneumothorax secondary to a penetrating injury, close the wound with a dressing sealed on three sides only to allow escape of air beneath the dressing. Insert a chest drain away from the wound and then close the dressing on the fourth side.

Different parameters must be used for athletes, those on medication such as beta-blocking agents and patients with fixed-rate pacemakers. In these patients the tachycardia may be less than you would expect for the blood volume lost. Infants and small children have different rate parameters for pulse, respiratory rate and blood pressure (Table 4.4).

For rapid volume replacement you must insert wide-bore, short-length cannulas into the cephalic vein at the wrist, the basocephalic vein in the antecubital fossa or the long saphenous vein at the ankle.

Circulation

Hypovolaemic shock secondary to blood loss or plasma loss in burns requires early recognition and vigorous correction. Insert two wide-bore cannulas (16 gauge or larger) and replace the estimated volume loss with warm crystalloid solution (Hartmann's or Ringer's lactate) and blood. Blood loss in the adult can be classified as shown in Table 4.3.

Class 1 haemorrhage   Insert two intravenous cannulas, take blood for urgent cross-matching and replace the estimated volume loss with crystalloid solution. Monitor clinical signs, including pulse and blood pressure, closely.

Class 2–4 haemorrhage   Start similar management as for Class 1, with greater volume replacement, and request a surgical opinion. Class 3 and 4 patients require vigorous fluid replacement, including immediate blood transfusion. Use O negative or type-specific blood and obtain an urgent surgical consultation with a view to early intervention.

Table 4.3   Classification of blood loss by volume and clinical signs in a normal adult

Class	Blood volume lost	Clinical signs
1	Up to 15% (750 ml)	Patient's skin is pale, pulse rate is increased but less than 100 beats/min; blood pressure is unchanged and capillary refill is normal (less than 2 s)
2	15–30% (750–1500 ml)	Skin is pale and patient is anxious; pulse rate is elevated to 100 beats/min and capillary refill is more than 2 s; systolic blood pressure is unchanged but diastolic pressure is elevated, leading to a narrow pulse pressure
3	30–40% (1.5–2 litres)	Patient is pale, sweaty and confused, with a tachycardia of 100 beats/min or more and blood pressure falling below 100 mmHg
4	40% (2 litres) or more	Patient is confused or unconscious with pale skin, a marked tachycardia of 140 beats/min or more and blood pressure falling below 70 mmHg

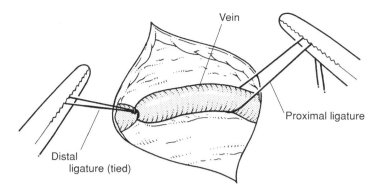

Fig. 4.3 Venous cutdown: exposed vein with distal ligation prior to cannulation.

Table 4.4 Normal observations of pulse and blood pressure in children (estimated average systolic blood pressure = 80 + age in years × 2)

	BP (systolic)	Pulse rate (/min)	Respiratory rate (/min)
Infant (<1 year)	80	160	40
Pre-school (1–5 years)	90	140	30
Adolescent (5–12 years)	100	120	20

Technique of venous cutdown   Use the long saphenous vein at the ankle. Other veins can be used, including, in an emergency, the long saphenous vein in the inguinal region. Apply a tourniquet above the ankle and clean the skin with antiseptic solution below and anterior to the medial malleolus. Cover the surrounding area with sterile towels. Infiltrate the skin 2 cm above and anterior to the medial malleolus with 2–3 ml of 1% lignocaine solution and make a 2–2.5 cm transverse incision. Identify the vein using blunt dissection of the subcutaneous tissues and free it along a length of approximately 2 cm. Pass two ligatures under the vein. Tie the lower ligature and leave the upper one untied (Fig. 4.3).

Hold both ligatures with forceps in opposition. Incise the vein with sharp scissors and dilate the venotomy with fine forceps before inserting a 16 gauge cannula. Finally, tie the proximal ligature and cut both (Fig. 4.4).

Connect the cannula to an intravenous infusion set. Close the skin with interrupted sutures, secure the distal tubing of the infusion set to the skin and cover the wound with a strong dressing.

> Avoid central lines where possible as the high flow-rates necessary for resuscitation cannot be achieved with long lines. Failure to cannulate the vein may occur in severe shock when vessels are neither visible nor palpable. Under these circumstances perform a venous cutdown.

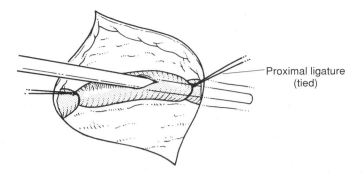

Fig. 4.4   Venous cutdown: placement of the cannula.

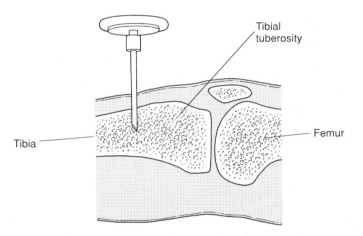

Fig. 4.5   Intraosseous needle placement in tibial marrow.

Intraosseous transfusion is the technique of choice for infants and children when cannulation of a vein is difficult. The preferred sites of infusion are the anterior surface of the uninjured tibia 2–3 cm below the tibial tuberosity or the anterolateral surface of the femur 3 cm above the lateral condyle. Clean the skin and infiltrate 1% lignocaine. Insert an intraosseous transfusion needle or a 16 gauge 1 cm bone marrow aspiration needle at 90° to the skin and advance it until a 'give' is felt on entering the marrow (Fig. 4.5).

Remove the stylette of the needle and attach a 5 ml syringe to the needle and aspirate marrow to confirm needle placement. Use 250 ml syringes to administer boluses of crystalloid fluid (20 ml/km) to the assessed volume of blood loss. Once the volume was has been corrected insert venous cannulas and withdraw the intraosseous needle.

Burns

Initial volume replacement in a patient with burns or scalds is estimated using the formula: half the body weight × percentage of body surface burned. Estimate the percentage area of burns from the observed partial- and full-thickness injuries but do not include areas of erythema of the skin. Give this initial volume of fluid over a 4-hour period, starting at the time of thermal injury. Subsequently follow local burns unit guidelines for fluid replacement (see also Chapter 9).

Cardiac tamponade

Penetrating injuries of the chest carry the risk of pericardial tamponade. Suspect this condition in chest injuries, particularly if the wound lies within the nipple line anteriorly or the medial border of the scapula posteriorly. Electromechanical disassociation complexes without output associated with poor-quality heart sounds should raise the suspicion of tamponade. Perform a cardiocentesis. Distended neck veins and pulsus paradoxus are not usually evident in hypovolaemic patients.

Technique of pericardiocentesis

Clean and drape the skin over the xiphisternum and left anterior costal margin. Infiltrate an area to the left and below the xiphoid cartilage with antiseptic solution. Ensure that the patient is connected to an ECG monitor. Attach a three-way tap 16 gauge cannula over a 15 cm or longer needle and 50 ml syringe. Insert the needle through the anaesthetized area and advance it at an angle of 45° towards the top of the left scapula. Aspirate the syringe continuously and watch the ECG monitor (Fig. 4.6). If an injury complex appears (ST/T wave changes or widened, enlarged QRS complexes) before blood is aspirated it is unlikely that tamponade is present.

If you aspirate blood without an injury complex you have performed a successful pericardiocentesis. It is unlikely that more than 25–30 ml of blood will be removed but you should observe a definite clinical improvement. After successful completion of the procedure transfer the patient to the operating theatre for emergency thoracotomy. Leave the cannula in place and perform further pericardiocentesis if clinically indicated.

> Do not advance the needle in the presence of an injury impulse on the ECG monitor as subsequent aspiration of blood will be from the cardiac chamber.

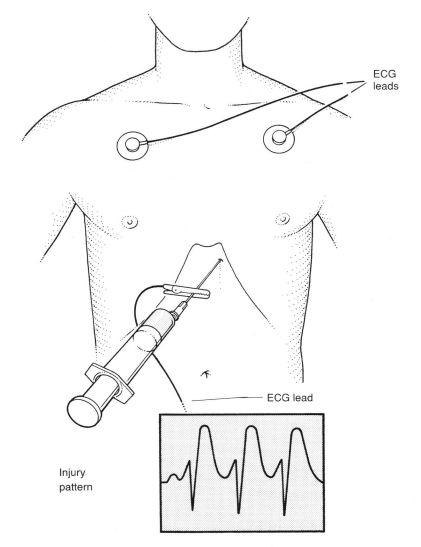

ECG
leads

ECG lead

Injury
pattern

Fig. 4.6 Pericardiocentesis.

Diagnostic peritoneal lavage (DPL)

During the secondary assessment of the patient for suspected abdominal injury, diagnostic peritoneal lavage may be required to eliminate intraperitoneal haemorrhage or hollow viscus injury. Perform this procedure early in an unstable hypovolaemic patient.

Technique of DPL

Catheterize the bladder and insert a naso- or orogastric tube. Clean and drape the abdomen and flanks. Use 5–10 ml of 1% lignocaine with adrenaline solution to anaesthetize the skin in the midline one-third of the way from the umbilicus to the symphysis pubis. Incise the skin vertically in the midline and separate the underlying subcutaneous tissues with skin retractors. Secure haemostasis with firm pressure.

Expose and incise the fascia and secure haemostasis. Apply two artery forceps to the exposed peritoneum, gently raise it and make a small hole with scissors in the peritoneal membrane. Insert a dialysis catheter into the peritoneal cavity and gently advance it towards the pelvis. Connect the catheter to a syringe. Aspiration of frank blood indicates a positive tap: arrange to transfer the patient to the theatre for formal laparotomy. If frank blood is not aspirated fix the catheter in place and attach an intravenous infusion set. Infuse 1 litre of warmed (37°C) normal saline into the peritoneal cavity (use 10 ml/kg in children). Leave the fluid in the peritoneal cavity for 5–10 min, depending on the patient's condition, then place the infusion bag on the floor to drain the saline from the peritoneal cavity. Send a sample of peritoneal fluid to the laboratory. The finding of 100 000 red blood cells or 500 white blood cells per cubic millimetre indicates a positive test. Observation of bacteria or vegetable fibres suggests perforation and laparotomy will be required.

> - Negative lavage does not exclude a retroperitoneal injury or diaphragmatic tear.
> - Be prepared for the thin abdominal wall in children and infants. Proceed with caution.

TREATMENT OF LOCALIZED INFECTION

Abscess

An abscess is a localized collection of pus, usually subcutaneous. Treat it by incision and drainage. When a digit is affected use a digital block with plain lignocaine (avoid adrenaline). General anaesthesia is required for other sites. The incision should be at least two-thirds of the width of the abscess to allow adequate drainage of pus. Promote drainage by the insertion of a short single length of ribbon gauze for 24 hours. Do not pack the abscess cavity as this prevents drainage and causes discomfort, particularly on removal.

> Do not delay incision when pain is present and sleep is disturbed.

Infected sebaceous cyst

Treat an infected sebaceous cyst by incision/drainage under local anaesthetic if it is small; otherwise use a general anaesthetic. Do not attempt to excise the capsule of the sebaceous cyst. After incision and

> Cover the punctum of the cyst prior to injection of local anaesthetic to prevent local anaesthetic and purulent material being expressed under force into your eye.

drainage refer the patient to his/her general practitioner with a view to subsequent elective complete excision of the cyst.

Paronychia

Paronychia is defined as pus around or adjacent to the nail. There is usually a tender area around the nail with increasing pain and swelling.

Treatment

Perform a ring block using 1% plain lignocaine. Make a longitudinal incision parallel to the nail (Fig. 4.7).

Take a swab for culture to determine sensitivity of the infecting organism. Apply a tulle gras dressing, put the hand in a sling and supply adequate analgesia. No antibiotic is indicated at this stage.

Pulp infection

Infection of the pulp of the finger leads to a swollen, painful, tender pulp of the finger. The patient gives a history that the pain is increasing and is of a throbbing nature that disturbs sleep.

Investigation

X-ray the finger to see if there is any involvement of the terminal phalanx. Perform a ring block using 1% plain lignocaine and make a

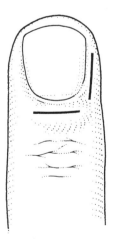

Fig. 4.7 Incision sites for paronychia. Site of incision may depend upon any collection of pus.

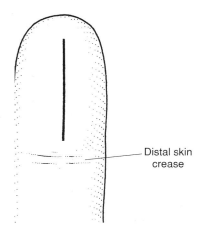

Fig. 4.8   Incision site for finger pulp infection.

longitudinal incision in the middle of the pulp. Make sure that the incision does not go beyond the distal crease (Fig. 4.8).

Do not delay incision and do not rely on antibiotic therapy as osteomyelitis of the distal phalanx may result.

Suturing technique

This is one of the most important surgical procedures undertaken in the Accident and Emergency Department. If the proper technique is not used the patient might end up with a permanent disfiguring scar. Most suturing in the Accident Department is done under local anaesthesia, usually with 1% plain lignocaine. Use a synthetic monofilament suture material (4/0–5/0).

Use absorbable material for subcutaneous sutures.

Technique

Clean the wound with aqueous chlorhexidine or normal saline. Remove any foreign body and irrigate with chlorhexidine or normal saline. Excise the margins of the wound if they are ragged. Approximate the wound edges and suture them carefully with interrupted sutures to appose the edges accurately (Chapter 1). If the suture line is under tension then mattress sutures should be applied. Cover the wound with a dry dressing and elevate the injured part for at least 12–24 hours. Give tetanus toxoid if the patient is not already immunized against tetanus or if immunity has lapsed or is in doubt. Give antibiotic if the wound is contaminated.

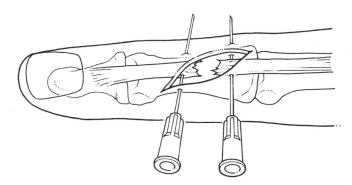

Fig. 4.9 Insertion of 'green' hypodermic needle for apposition extensor tendon repair.

Extensor tendon laceration

Laceration (division) of a single extensor tendon is diagnosed by inability to extend the finger. Injury may be closed or open. Division of the extensor tendon usually occurs in elderly patients; an open cut extensor tendon is caused by a sharp object going through the skin over the extensor tendon.

Technique of repair

Under digital block (1% plain lignocaine) clean the wound and explore it. Use a finger tourniquet to achieve a bloodless field in young patients but if the patient is elderly avoid a finger tourniquet. Identify the proximal and distal cut ends of the tendon(s). Stabilize the cut tendons by passing a 19 gauge hypodermic needle through the skin and tendon, keeping the finger in extension. Suture the tendon with non-absorbable suture material (Fig. 4.9).

Apply a dry dressing and immobilize the finger in a Zimmer splint. Give antibiotic cover if the wound is contaminated.

> Do not use lignocaine with adrenaline for digital anaesthesia. If there are multiple tendon injuries to the tendons of the thumb or flexor injuries, the patient should be admitted for formal exploration and repair.

DISLOCATIONS

Shoulder

This usually occurs after a fall on to the outstretched hand with the arm in rotation. A shoulder dislocation may be anterior or posterior, subcoracoid or intrathoracic, causing severe discomfort and restriction of joint movement. On palpation there is a depression over the anterior shoulder joint.

Treatment

Successful reduction can be achieved with gentle manipulation under intravenous sedation and analgesia, with additional oxygen and recorded pulse oximetry.

Hippocratic manipulation   Apply traction against countertraction in the axilla. The operator's stockinged foot is placed in the axilla, palpating the head of the humerus, and helps with the reduction. (This technique is rarely used.)

Kocher's manipulation   Use this method, which is more convenient than the Hippocratic manipulation. Lie the patient supine on a couch and stand on the affected side. Flex the elbow to 90° and hold the wrist in one hand and the humerus above the elbow in the other. Apply gentle traction to the humerus and maintain the traction. Gently rotate the humerus laterally by moving the forearm out through 50–60°. Hold the limb in external rotation and bring the elbow forward and medially to the front of the chest. At the same time rotate the humerus medially by bringing the hand over to the opposite shoulder. All the above movements should be done slowly and gently. After the manipulation maintain the final position and place a soft cotton wool pad in the axilla. Apply body bandages to hold the arm against the chest.

> - Check and record limb sensation and circulation before and after manipulation.
> - Always obtain X-rays before and after manipulation.
> - Review the patient the following day.

Patella

Diagnosis

Take a careful history as half the cases may have a predisposing factor. A dislocation usually occurs when the thigh muscles are relaxed. Any forceful pressure over the medial side of the patella can result in a lateral dislocation.
    Obtain skyline X-rays before manipulation to detect any fracture.

Manipulation

Under nitrous oxide and oxygen or intravenous sedation place the palm of your hand over the lateral aspect of the patella. Apply gentle upward and medial force and the patella will reduce. Immobilize the knee in a plaster backslab or Robert Jones bandage.

Knee

Dislocation of the knee is usually due to direct injury to the upper end of the tibia and can also occur due to hyperextension and a twisting

The popliteal artery can be damaged with obvious or delayed circulatory changes in the distal limb. Obtain preoperative and postoperative X-rays. Record the neurovascular findings at the foot and ankle and record the stability of the joint. Immobilize the knee in a plaster cylinder and admit the patient.

injury to the knee. The tibia is usually posteriorly dislocated. The injury should be suspected from the mechanism of injury and the visible deformity of the joint. Prior to manipulation, test and record peripheral circulation and obtain knee-joint X-rays.

Manipulation under general anaesthesia

Apply gentle traction with direct pressure over the upper tibia posteriorly to correct the deformity. Check the peripheral circulation and record your findings. Immobilize the knee in an above-knee plaster of Paris slab. Obtain X-rays after manipulation and admit the patient to orthopaedic care.

Fingers

Hyperextension or flexion injury can cause dislocation of the metacarpophalangeal, proximal or distal interphalangeal joint.

Treatment

Use nitrous oxide and oxygen or a digital nerve block to obtain adequate analgesia. Reduce the dislocation by traction and apply garter strapping to fix the injured digit to the next finger. Obtain X-rays after manipulation to confirm reduction. Elevate the hand in a high sling and prescribe analgesia. Review the patient the next day. If the joint is stable, garter strapping is sufficient. If the joint is unstable the patient should be admitted for repair of the collateral ligament.

Ankle

Abduction or external rotation can cause dislocation of the ankle. If the force of injury continues it may lead to fracture and dislocation of the ankle. The dislocation is usually very obvious because of deformity, swelling and pain. Dislocation of the ankle is an emergency that should be dealt with immediately, as delay may cause skin necrosis. Do not wait for X-rays to confirm the diagnosis: act at once.

Treatment

Under nitrous oxide and oxygen or intravenous sedation and analgesia apply gentle traction to the os calcis. With simultaneous pressure over the lateral malleolus, apply pressure in an upward direction to correct the deformity.

Record the stability of the joint and the presence of peripheral circulation. Immobilize the ankle in a below-knee plaster of Paris slab and obtain check X-rays after reduction. Admit the patient for elevation and observation.

WRIST FRACTURES

The most common wrist injury is a Colles fracture. It appears in the elderly and is associated with a fall on to the outstretched hand. Pain, swelling and a 'dinner-fork' deformity are suggestive of a fracture. The fracture is usually transverse across the distal radius, usually within a centimetre of the carpal radial joint. The fracture may be comminuted, may involve the articular surface and may be associated with a fracture of the lower ulna or ulnar styloid.

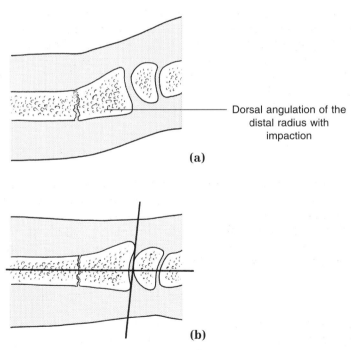

Dorsal angulation of the distal radius with impaction

(a)

(b)

Fig. 4.10 Colles fracture. **(a)** Lateral X-ray before manipulation. **(b)** Target for successful manipulation.

Deformity (Fig. 4.10) is due to:

- the impaction of the distal radius into the proximal shaft;
- dorsal angulation of the distal fragment;
- dorsal angulation and radial deviation of the lower radius.

Manipulation

Manipulation is undertaken under general anaesthesia or Bier's block. Roll a stockinette support over the forearm to the elbow. Ask your assistant to stabilize the upper forearm and apply traction to the arm and hand to correct the impaction. Then correct the dorsal angulation by flexion of the wrist and pressure over the distal radius, flexing the wrist to approximately 30–40°. At the same time overcome the radial deformity by placing the flexed wrist in approximately 10° of ulnar deviation. While maintaining the corrected position roll the stockinette down from just below the elbow to the metacarpophalangeal joints of the fingers. Apply a thin layer of wool around the wrist. Finally, apply a below-elbow backslab to encompass the radial and dorsal surfaces of the forearm and wrist, extending from below the cubital fossa to the metacarpophalangeal joints of the fingers. Roll the stockinette back over the plaster edges and manipulate the plaster firmly over the wrist to maintain traction and

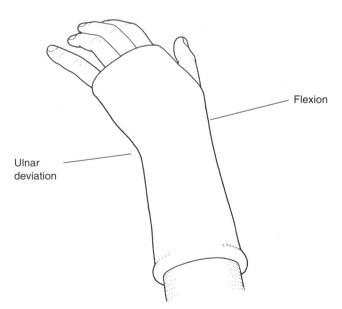

Flexion

Ulnar deviation

Fig. 4.11   Colles fracture: POP back slab.

ulnar deviation. Secure the plaster with a cotton elasticized bandage (Fig. 4.11).

Maintain anaesthesia until you have a check X-ray to ensure that impaction and deformity have been corrected. If the reduction has been unsuccessful further manipulation is possible. Once the position is acceptable the patient can be allowed to recover from the anaesthetic and may be discharged home with the arm supported in a sling. Prescribe analgesia and give plaster maintenance instructions. An outpatient appointment should be made for the Orthopaedic review clinic and completion of the plaster on the following day.

Greenstick or buckle-type fractures of the lower radius in infants and small children rarely require manipulation. They can be managed satisfactorily by the application of a dorsal plaster slab and referral the next day for an orthopaedic opinion.

Smith's fracture, which is a reverse of the Colles deformity, is an unstable fracture. Seek an orthopaedic opinion before devising a management plan.

- Check the elbow joint for injury before manipulation of the wrist.
- Check for signs of medial nerve compression before manipulation.
- If there is an abrasion or break in the skin, this requires prescription of an appropriate antibiotic.
- A Bier's block is a two-person procedure with the anaesthetist responsible for the block and the maintenance of the cuff. The Accident Officer is responsible for the manipulation of the fracture.

General notes on plaster technique

- Plastering is indicated to immobilize a fracture. After reduction of a dislocation apply only a plaster slab in the Accident and Emergency Department. If the patient is admitted to hospital then a complete plaster may be applied. In this case you should split the plaster to minimize compression and distal swelling.
- The plaster should immobilize the joint above and below the fracture site (except for a Colles fracture).
- Immobilize joints in the anatomical position.
- The plaster should be reviewed after 24 hours with a view to completing it.
- Protect bony prominences with adequate wool prior to application of the plaster.

NOTE: LOCAL GUIDELINES

When you perform any of the practical procedures described, you must follow departmental guidelines. Do not attempt them until you have been formally instructed, and have your initial efforts supervised by an experienced member of medical staff.

Orthopaedic surgery

5

Hugh J. Clarke

This chapter has been designed to give a trainee surgeon the basic approaches to common operations that may be seen during basic surgical training. These have been grouped into regions of the locomotor system.

UPPER LIMB

Carpal tunnel syndrome

Anaesthetic

Use local anaesthesia with 5 ml of lignocaine 2% (no adrenaline) or a general anaesthetic.

Position

Place the patient supine, with the arm extended on a hand table. Apply a pneumatic tourniquet.

Approach

Make a midline skin incision from the distal transverse crease to 4 cm distal in the midline to the ulnar border of the palmaris longus tendon. Deepen the incision strictly in the midline down to the transverse carpal ligament. Continue the development through the whole length of the incision (Fig. 5.1).

Use a strong, self-retaining retractor to give increased exposure and reduce any haemorrhage. Make a small incision through the thick transverse carpal ligament until a small perforation is achieved. Next slide a McDonald's dissector proximally to guard the median nerve. Continue the incision through the transverse carpal ligament under direct vision with either a scalpel or scissors. After full decompression proximally carry the incision distally. The median nerve lies directly under the completed incision and should be inspected throughout its length (Fig. 5.2).

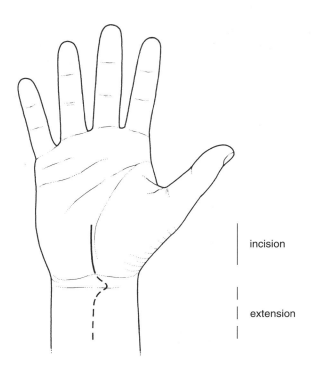

incision

extension

Fig. 5.1 Midline skin incision to approach the carpal tunnel.

The main risk is damage to the median nerve and its motor branch. Always visualize and identify the structures to be incised. The palmar branch of the median nerve divides in the proximal radial side of the wound. All incisions should be strictly in the midline. Wound extension proximal to the distal wrist crease should be done in a Z fashion to avoid skin contracture (Fig. 5.1).

Closure

Use skin sutures only.

De Quervain's release

Anaesthetic

Use 2% lignocaine in the line of the skin incision or general anaesthetic.

Position

Place the patient supine with the arm extended on an arm table. Apply a tourniquet after exsanguination.

Approach

Make a lazy S skin incision. A transverse incision is more cosmetic although access is poorer (Fig. 5.3).

After the skin incision, use blunt dissection to identify the superficial radial nerve, which runs along the line of the skin incision towards the anatomical snuff box. Mobilize and preserve the nerve. Identify the dorsal ligament directly under the branches of the nerve. Flex and extend the thumb with abduction to identify the areas of the tendon and of the ligament. Incise through the first dorsal compartment and continue the release proximally and distally to expose the tendon throughout the length of the incision. Lift the individual ten-

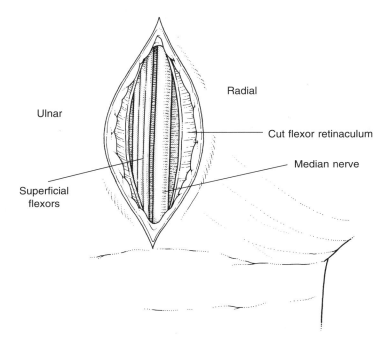

Ulnar

Radial

Cut flexor retinaculum

Median nerve

Superficial flexors

Fig. 5.2   Dissection of the carpal tunnel, showing the median nerve.

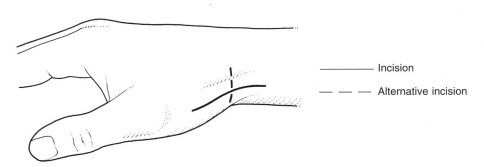

———— Incision

— — — Alternative incision

Fig. 5.3   Lazy S skin incision used in De Quervain's release.

dons with a tendon hook to check that they have been fully released and identify the adductor pollicis longus tendon and the extensor pollicis brevis tendon in their bed (Fig. 5.4).

Skin closure

Use fine interrupted monofilament or subcuticular sutures.

Release of deep flexor tendon trigger finger

Anaesthetic

Use 2% lignocaine in the line of skin incision and midline of the metacarpal (no adrenaline) or general anaesthetic.

Position

Place the patient supine with the arm extended on an arm table. Use an exsanguinating tourniquet.

Approach

For the lateral three rays make a transverse skin incision 0.5 cm distal to the distal transverse skin crease. For the index finger use the line of the skin crease. Deepen the superficial skin incision using blunt dissection with scissors in a longitudinal direction strictly in the midline of the digit (Fig. 5.5).

> • Dissect carefully after the skin incision to preserve all branches of the superficial radial nerve.
> • There is a large anatomical variation of the abductor and extensor brevis tendons. If full movements are not obtained on testing the tendons with a tendon hook, consider whether there may be a further tendon sheath requiring decompression.

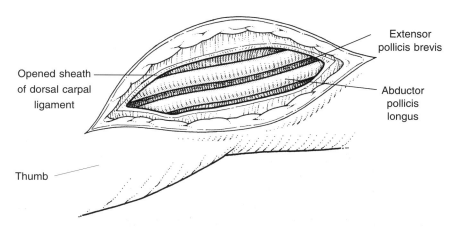

Extensor
pollicis brevis

Opened sheath
of dorsal carpal
ligament

Abductor
pollicis
longus

Thumb

Fig. 5.4 De Quervain's release.

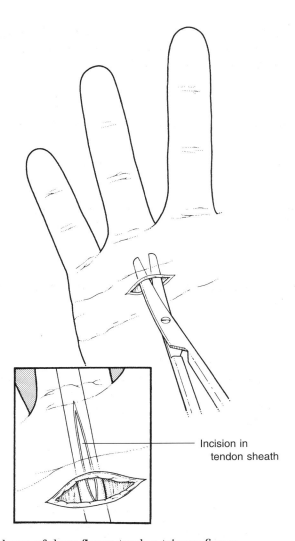

Incision in
tendon sheath

Fig. 5.5   Release of deep flexor tendon trigger finger.

Expose the flexor sheath with small Langenbeck retractors placed proximally and distally. Make a small incision through the flexor sheath taking care not to enter the tendon on its deep surface. Use small-bladed scissors to enlarge this incision proximally and distally to completely release the flexor sheath up to the flexor crease at the base of the finger. Passively flex and extend the distal finger to check full excursion of the deep tendon.

> During dissection the digital nerves to the ray are only a few millimetres away from the midline. Always use blunt dissection after the skin incision and keep to the midline of the ray. Check that the flexor sheath has been well decompressed distally through this proximal wound.

Closure

Close only the skin with fine interrupted sutures.

Ganglion

Indications

This common tumour of the hand may arise from the synovial joints; it is commonly associated with tendon sheaths and occasionally can arise directly from bone or tendon. The hand is the commonest site for these benign tumours, which are often sited over the dorsum of the wrist or on the volar surface adjacent to the radial artery. The general principles of excision remain the same, independent of the anatomical site. Surgical excision offers the highest rate of cure.

Anaesthetic

Remove dorsal ganglions under local anaesthetic; tumours sited around the radial artery may be more easily removed under general anaesthetic.

Position

Place the patient supine with a hand table.

Approach

- **Dorsal site**: Make a transverse skin incision in the Langer's lines. After the skin incision identify the capsule and develop the plane around the ganglion to reach its base. It is important to take a reasonable margin of tissue surrounding the origin of the ganglion to try to prevent recurrence.
- **Radial artery site**: Make a longitudinal incision under tourniquet just radial to the flexor carpi radialis. Using blunt dissection, fully identify the artery before removal of the ganglion. Small vessels may be ligated overlying the ganglion preserving the main radial artery. Excise all loculations where possible down to the base of the carpus, where the tumour arises.

> - It is important to excise a reasonable margin of tissue from the base of the lesion to avoid recurrence.
> - Surgical complications are dependent on the surrounding anatomical structures.

Skin closure

Close the skin with fine interrupted monofilament or subcuticular sutures.

Release of tennis elbow (extensor epicondylitis)

Anaesthetic

Use a general anaesthetic or regional block.

Position

Place the patient supine with an exsanguinating tourniquet in place. Flex the arm up to 90° with the lateral epicondyle facing you.

Make a curved incision from the lateral epicondylar ridge of the humerus in line with the radial head 2 cm distal to the radial head (Fig. 5.6).

Deepen the skin incision with blunt dissection to gain access to the epicondyle. The primary muscle to be released is the extensor carpi radialis brevis with its aponeurosis off the epicondyle. Release this in a V fashion from the epicondyle with excision of a small amount of the insertion. The extensor carpi radialis longus muscle inserts on to the epicondylar ridge and should be released in the line along the epicondylar ridge. Remove any degenerate tendon at the common extensor origin. If necessary, trim the bony epicondyle (Fig. 5.7).

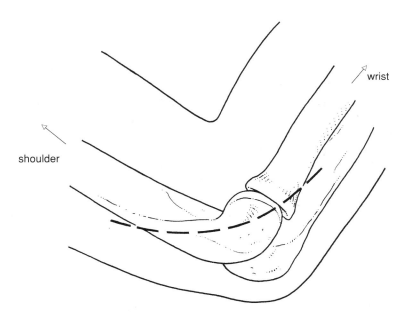

Fig. 5.6 Incision for the release of tennis elbow.

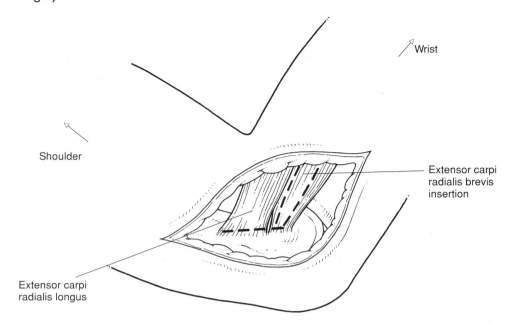

Fig. 5.7 Release of tennis elbow (extensor epicondylitis).

> Do not take the deep incision further than 2 cm distal to the radial head to prevent damage to the posterior interosseous nerve.

Closure

Close the V incision in a Y fashion to shorten the common extensor origin. Use absorbable sutures. Close the skin with subcuticular or fine interrupted monofilament sutures. Immobilize the arm in a broad arm sling for 3 weeks.

LOWER LIMB

There are many approaches to the hip. The majority of operations can be accomplished through either the modified lateral or the posterior approach.

Modified lateral approach

Anaesthetic

Use a general anaesthetic or regional anaesthetic with a spinal/epidural block.

Position

Place the patient either supine or lateral. The lateral position requires less assistance. Place suitable anterior supports on the pubis or anterior superior iliac spines and over the sacrum. Provide support for the ipsilateral arm. Protect pressure areas with padded wool under the lateral popliteal nerve, the ankle and the arms.

Approach

Make a straight incision over the greater trochanter with equal limbs proximally and distally with a gentle posterior curve to the proximal incision (Fig. 5.8).

Incise the fascia lata in the line of the skin incision and split the gluteus maximus muscle in the line of its fibres. Identify the broad band of the gluteus medius tendon inserting into the superior and anterior greater trochanter. Insert a pair of curved Mayo scissors underneath this large tendon and remove it with sharp dissection or cutting diathermy leaving a portion of tendon attached to the trochanter and a portion attached to the anterior third of the gluteus medius muscle (Fig. 5.9).

Reflect the anterior gluteus anteriorly, including the small gluteus minimus muscle which you will find beneath it. The plane of dissection should be along the hip capsule. Use a square Holman retractor inserted carefully over the lip of the acetabulum to reflect the muscle.

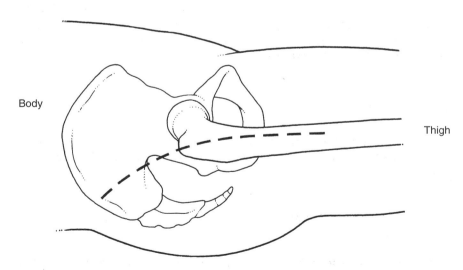

Body

Thigh

Fig. 5.8 Modified lateral approach to the hip: initial incision.

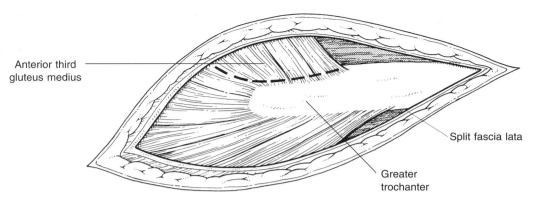

Anterior third
gluteus medius

Split fascia lata

Greater
trochanter

Fig. 5.9 Modified lateral approach to the hip: deep incision.

- The sciatic nerve runs posterior to the greater trochanter. Do not identify this in the modified lateral incision unless any dissection is planned for this area.
- Place retractors underneath the gluteus medius muscle (to reflect it anteriorly) directly on the capsule, to prevent damage to the femoral nerve.
- It is vitally important to maintain tendon on each side of the cut gluteus medius in order to obtain secure closure of the gluteus medius tendon.

Closure

Close the wound in layers with No. 1 synthetic absorbable sutures. Skin closure: as required. Use one deep and one superficial vacuum drain.

Posterior approach

Position

Place the patient in the lateral position using support as described for the modified lateral approach. Place the posterior support higher on to the sacrum or lumbar spine area to allow the posterior extension of the proximal wound. Make a lateral incision starting 10 cm distal to the greater trochanter and extending posteriorly and superiorly towards the posterior superior iliac spine (Fig. 5.10).

Incise the iliotibial band in the line of the skin incision and split the gluteus maximus fibres in the same line. Using blunt dissection with the full hand, reflect the posterior muscles off the posterior trochanter. Flex the lower leg to 90° and internally rotate it with adduction to reveal the external rotators inserting into the inter-trochanteric crest. At this stage you must identify the sciatic nerve to check its position in relation to the acetabulum. When you have protected the nerve, insert curved Mayo scissors underneath the short external rotators just inferior to the posterior insertion of the gluteus medius tendon. Divide these tendons by sharp dissection or cutting diathermy to control the vessels anastomosing around the intertrochanteric crest (Fig. 5.11).

Using a swab, reflect them off the capsule to reveal the whole posterior hip joint. Access to the joint can now be made through the chosen capsular incision.

Closure

Reattachment of the external rotators is not essential. Close the iliotibial tract with strong synthetic absorbable sutures and use a standard superficial closure over vacuum drains.

The sciatic nerve runs close to the external rotators. You must identify it throughout a reasonable length prior to incising the external rotators. Maintain caution throughout the operative procedure, particularly when excising the posterior capsule of the joint to make sure that the position of the nerve has not altered.

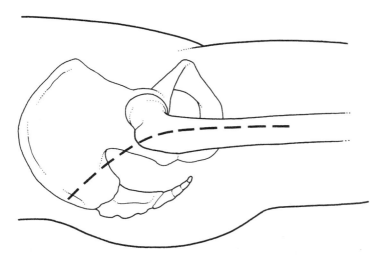

Fig. 5.10 Posterior approach to the hip: initial incision.

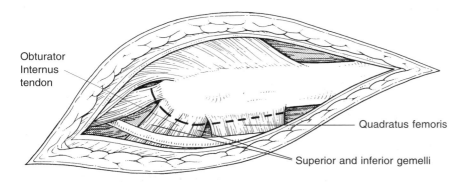

Obturator Internus tendon

Quadratus femoris

Superior and inferior gemelli

Fig. 5.11 Posterior approach to the hip: division of the tendons.

Hemiarthroplasty

Indications

Hemiarthroplasty is required for displaced fractured neck of femur in the elderly patient, where there is a high risk of vascular necrosis.

Approach

The patient should be placed in the lateral position. While this operation can be performed through either a modified lateral or posterior approach we prefer the modified lateral approach as there is a high risk of dislocation through a posterior approach, particularly in the confused or parkinsonian patient.

Capsular incision After you have reflected the gluteus medius anteriorly, incise the anterior capsule and excise it in a T fashion to gain access to the remaining neck of femur. Clear the neck with a periosteal elevator and place a Holman retractor under the inferior medial and superolateral neck. Place a trial hemiarthroplasty prosthesis on the anterior surface of the femur with the centre of the head opposite the superior trochanter. Mark the femoral neck with an osteotome prior to sectioning. Section the neck with an oscillating saw, being careful to maintain a neutral angle on the neck (Fig. 5.12).
  You now have access to the head of the femur. Incise the capsule fully on to the lip of the acetabulum to allow full exposure of the head. Insert two corkscrews through the fracture into the head to give good purchase. Extract the head by traction and leverage assisted by a skid behind the femoral head. The acetabulum is now exposed; excise the remaining ligamentum teres. Clear any remaining fragments from the acetabulum.

Preparation of the femur You may use either an uncemented hemiarthroplasty, e.g. Austin Moore prosthesis, or a cemented one, e.g. Thompson's prosthesis. First ream the femur by taking a small portion out of the neck laterally to allow access for the reamers. Place a narrow, blunt bone-spike into the centre of the femur to identify the centre of the canal. Then insert to the hilt a broach corresponding to the designed prosthesis. Measure the femoral head using circumferential gauges and identify the correct-sized prosthesis (actual size or one size smaller). Then insert the definitive prosthesis with the collar placed on to the calcar of the neck by direct impaction with a polythene-headed punch. Reduce the hip by internal rotation with traction in an axial direction. Check the stability of the prosthesis in external rotation with adduction and check complete reduction.

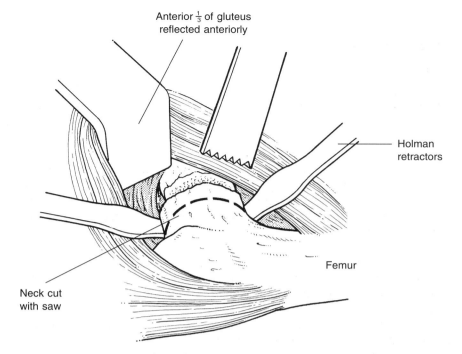

Anterior ⅓ of gluteus
reflected anteriorly

Holman
retractors

Femur

Neck cut
with saw

Fig. 5.12   Neck of the femur exposed for saw cut.

Close the wound in layers, with particular attention to the secure closure of the gluteus medius with interrupted synthetic absorbable sutures and standard interrupted closure of the remaining layers over vacuum drains.

> In general, precautions are as described for the modified lateral approach. Pay rigorous attention to antisepsis and use prophylactic antibiotics.

Dynamic hip screw

Indications

Intertrochanteric fractured neck of femur.

Anaesthetic

Use general anaesthesia or regional spinal/epidural block.

Position

Place the patient in the supine position on a fracture reduction table with full abduction of the contralateral limb and a straight to mildly abducted affected limb. Place an image intensifier to obtain full excursion through an AP and lateral X-ray of the hip including the superior head of the femur. Place the ipsilateral arm across the chest to allow access to the top end of the femur. Use a sterile exclusion drape to allow access only to the top of the femur.

Approach

Make a direct lateral incision through the skin extending from the greater trochanter to the required distance inferiorly for the length of plate desired. Make a straight lateral incision through the iliotibial band. Cut the vastus lateralis along its posterior margin leaving a small cuff of posterior tissue and reflect the muscle anteriorly off the femur to give access to the shaft. Clean the shaft with a periosteal elevator. Under image-intensifier control first place a guide wire on the anterior neck using a standard valgus angle guide to give a wire placement in the centre of the neck on the AP X-ray projection. Make a drill hole in the lateral cortex to allow placement of the guide wire in the same position on the AP plane (Fig. 5.13).

Before you fully drill this wire, take an X-ray in the lateral plane to confirm central placement in both planes. Place the guide wire up to the subchondral bone. Check the length with the manufacturer's measuring device, set the triple reamer to the desired setting and select the screw length. Place the triple reamer over the guide wire and drill under image intensifier control up to the subchondral bone. (It is important to obtain images in both planes during this procedure.) In hard bone use a screw tap to cut the screw thread. Insert

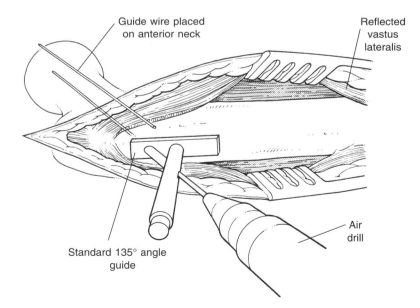

Fig. 5.13 Lateral approach for dynamic hip screw.

the definitive screw to the subchondral plate. Next insert an angled barrelled plate over the screw until it engages the cortex of the lateral femur. Secure this in place with the desired number of screws and insert a compression screw through the barrel into the sliding hip screw. Close the wound in layers with synthetic absorbable sutures and normal skin closure over vacuum drains.

Knee arthrotomy

The majority of major operations of the knee joint can be performed through a modification of the medial parapatellar incision, including arthroplasty, removal of loose bodies, synovectomy and reconstructive surgery.

Anaesthetic

Use a general or regional anaesthetic with an exsanguinating tourniquet placed high on the thigh.

Position

Supine.

Approach

Make a midline skin incision down through the superficial fascia. Reflect the incision medially to gain access to the capsule on the medial border of the patella. Make a curving incision 1 cm medial to the patella extending inferiorly the same distance medial to the patellar tendon. The incision through the synovium now gives full access to the knee joint. Extensive exposure can be obtained to cruciate ligaments, medial and lateral condyles by longitudinal incision of the quadriceps tendon and everting the patella prior to flexing the knee joint.

Closure

Close the fibrous capsule using thick, synthetic absorbable interrupted sutures. Carefully close the superficial layers.

Lesser toes – phalangeal fusions

Indications

Hammer and claw toe deformities.

- The guide wire must be inserted in the centre of the neck in both planes. If reduction is difficult before insertion, insert the guide wire freehand up the middle of the neck in both planes and ignore all angle guides. Reduce the fracture after insertion of the screw by placing the plate over the screw and using reduction clamps to bring this down into position on the femur.
- Radiographic control is essential throughout the guide-wire placement, triple reaming and screw insertion to prevent penetration of the femoral head.

- Take care of the skin at all times, as the poor blood supply to this area may result in poor wound healing. Keep to a minimum any undermining of the skin edges.
- Leave a reasonable cuff of fibrous capsule attached to the patella to allow secure closure.
- Use slowly absorbing sutures to allow strong healing prior to full absorption.
- Take care in the inferior part of the incision not to incise through the menisci or patellar tendon.
- Do not extend the distal skin incision over the tibial tubercle, as this may result in a tender scar on kneeling.

Anaesthetic

Use a local anaesthetic ring block/regional block or general anaesthetic.

Approach

Make an elliptical transverse full-thickness incision down to the PIP joint, excising an ellipse of the extensor tendon. Expose the condyles and release the collateral ligaments using a small-bladed knife inserted into the joint and slid up the side of the condyles. After mobilization, excise the condyles of the proximal joint with bone-cutters to give a flat surface in 90° planes to the bone. Excise the distal joint with a sharp osteotome used as a scraper, or nibblers. Fix the joint using a K-wire inserted through the centre of the phalanx (Fig. 5.14).

Ensure that you have good apposition of the joint surfaces and correct alignment of the toe at the end of the procedure. Mobility of the MTP joint should be checked. Bend the end of the K-wire to prevent migration.

> Keep the skin incision on the dorsal surface to prevent risk to the neurovascular bundles.

Closure

Use interrupted non-absorbable sutures to the skin. Remove the K-wires at 6 weeks.

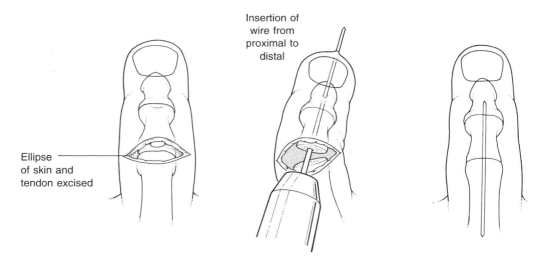

Insertion of wire from proximal to distal

Ellipse of skin and tendon excised

Fig. 5.14 Phalangeal fusion.

Achilles tendon repair

Indications

Complete rupture of the Achilles tendon in young athletes.

Anaesthetic

Use a general anaesthetic with tourniquet exsanguination.

Position

Position the patient prone or lateral with the affected limb uppermost.

Approach

Make a midline incision slightly to the medial side of the tendon and curve it away from the Achilles tendon in its distal portion. Directly after skin incision divide the paratenon and preserve and reflect it medially and laterally. Identify the ragged ruptured ends of the tendon and plantarflex the foot to approximate the ends. Repair the tendon using a Kessler type of repair using synthetic absorbable large sutures (Fig. 5.15).

Closure

Approximate the paratendon using fine absorbable sutures and carefully close the skin using interrupted or subcuticular sutures.

Apply plaster of Paris in plantarflexion with a backslab or a full split plaster.

> The main risk is to the sural nerve which lies lateral to the Achilles tendon. The posteromedial neurovascular bundle is placed well anterior but should be considered throughout the dissection. Make the skin incision to one side of the tendon to avoid rubbing shoewear directly posteriorly.

Keller's first metatarsophalangeal arthroplasty

Indications

Severe hallux valgus or hallux rigidus in the elderly.

Anaesthetic

Use a general anaesthetic or local block.

Position

Prone.

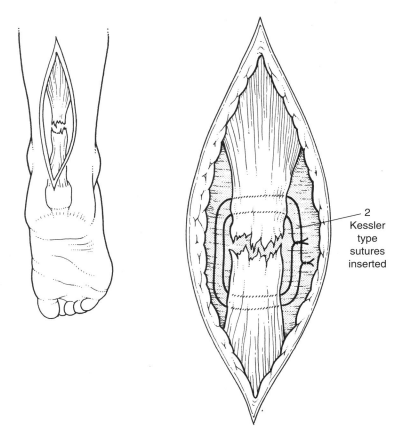

Fig. 5.15 Achilles tendon repair.

Procedure

Make a dorsomedial incision over the metatarsophalangeal joint extending on to the proximal phalanx. Preserve the extensor hallucis longus tendon. Reflect the capsule on the dorsal and volar sides of the bunion area and remove the bunion with a 1 inch osteotome, preserving the main MTP joint surface. Divide the proximal phalanx using an oscillating saw to remove 30% of the length of the proximal phalanx (Fig. 5.16).

Close the dorsomedial capsule using interrupted synthetic absorbable sutures. Use a standard skin closure. Postoperatively, plaster immobilization is not required.

First metatarsal osteotomy – Mitchell's

Indications

Symptomatic hallux valgus in younger patients.

Anaesthetic

Use a general or regional anaesthetic.

Position

Place the patient supine and apply an exsanguinating tourniquet.

Approach

Make a dorsomedial incision through the skin and preserve the dorsal digital nerve to the hallux. Make a longitudinal incision through the capsule and mobilize the capsule fully off the medial

- In severe hallux valgus full correction may not be easy. Before starting the procedure make a Y/V capsular incision to reef the medial capsule.
- Remove sufficient proximal phalanx to obtain correction.
- The dorsal digital nerves may be injured in the procedure. If this occurs, section the nerve rather than allowing neuroma formation.
- Further correction may be obtained in severe cases by release of the adductor hallucis tendon on the lateral border of the phalanx and Z-lengthening of the extensor hallucis longus. Ask for senior advice if you think this is necessary.

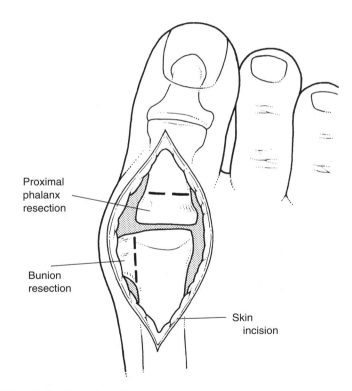

Proximal phalanx resection

Bunion resection

Skin incision

Fig. 5.16   Keller's arthroplasty.

border of the metatarsal. Preserve the extensor hallucis longus tendon on the proximal phalanx. Flex the toe to gain full access and place bone levers on the dorsal and plantar surfaces of the metatarsal. Remove the bunion with an osteotome, preserving the main articular surface of the MTP joint. Make two drill holes in the metatarsal, the distal one to the medial side and the proximal one to the lateral side of the metatarsal, with a gap of 7 mm between the two. Make the first osteotomy distally through three-quarters of the phalanx in a transverse plane. Make the second osteotomy 2 mm more proximally through the full phalanx and then remove the sliver of bone in between the two cuts with an osteotome. This leaves a small spike attached to the distal part of the metatarsal, which should be locked over the proximal phalanx (Fig. 5.17).

Pass a suture through the two holes and secure it to allow lateral displacement of the metatarsal head. Close the capsule securely using synthetic absorbable sutures.

Closure

Close the skin with non-absorbable interrupted sutures. Apply a plaster of Paris cast for 6 weeks.

(a)

(b)

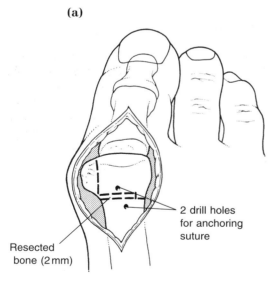
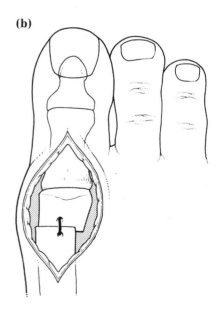

2 drill holes for anchoring suture

Resected bone (2 mm)

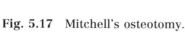

Fig. 5.17 Mitchell's osteotomy.

Skeletal traction pins

Indication

Traction pins are usually inserted into the upper tibia for control of a femoral fracture or through the calcaneum for tibial fractures. The Denham threaded pin is usually used for the upper tibia but for the calcaneum a smooth Steinman pin is preferable to prevent the creation of a hole within cancellous bone with movement of the calcaneum.

Anaesthetic

Use 20 ml of plain lignocaine. If manipulation of an acute fracture is necessary use a general anaesthetic.

Position

Place the patient supine and approach from the lateral side of the affected leg.

Tibial pin

Inject local anaesthetic 2 cm inferiorly and 1 cm posteriorly to the tibial tuberosity. Also inject anaesthetic on the opposite side, where the pin is expected to penetrate directly on to the periosteum. First insert the pin into a hand chuck, if the patient is elderly, but in a younger patient a low-speed, high-torque power drill is usually more satisfactory. Direct the pin at 90° to the axis of the tibial shaft and at 90° to the plane of the second toe pointing vertically. After the pin has been inserted the threads contact the outer cortex. Make six turns to engage the threads into the tibial cortex.

Calcaneal pin

Insert a calcaneal pin 3 cm below and 2 cm behind the tip of the lateral malleolus into the centre of the posterior of the calcaneum.

- In children with an open tibial tuberosity epiphysis insert the pin well away from the growth plate to prevent damage.
- It is essential that the plane of the pin is in the correct axis for good axial traction.
- Make sure that the pin is well anterior to the fibula to prevent any possible damage to the lateral popliteal nerve.

- Ensure you obtain correct alignment of the pin, as this is critical to applying good axial traction for a fractured tibia.
- Most neurovascular structures are well away from this insertion site.

Head injury and related neurosurgical techniques

6

Dorothy A. Lang and Peter Lees

MEDICAL PROBLEMS AND THEIR MANAGEMENT

Head injury is a leading cause of death in children and young adults. Remember that, in order to achieve a good outcome – or the best possible outcome given the severity of the brain damage – your patient requires:

- effective initial resuscitation in the field;
- rapid diagnosis and treatment in Accident and Emergency/primary surgical unit;
- appropriate neurosurgical referral;
- neurosurgical intensive care.

Head-injured patients tend to be in one of three categories:

- isolated head injury + intracranial mass lesion;
- isolated head injury + no intracranial mass lesion;
- head injury + multiple injuries ± intracranial mass lesion.

This chapter focuses on the management of head injury not complicated by intracranial mass lesions. The brain-injured patient who does not have an intracranial mass lesion has sustained either **focal** or **diffuse** brain damage (Table 6.1). In the reality of the clinical setting many patients have both focal and diffuse brain damage.

Diagnosis and initial management

The goals of initial management are to prevent/reverse secondary insults to the injured brain and to provide a milieu for recovery of dysfunctional/damaged brain. These goals are achieved by rapid resuscitation and by avoidance of hypotension and hypoxia (Table 6.2).

Options for initial management

After initial assessment and resuscitation, you must decide whether to discharge the patient, to admit to a primary surgical service for

Table 6.1   Types of brain damage after head injury

Focal lesions include:
- Haematomas
- Cerebral contusions
- Lesions due to elevated intracranial pressure (ICP)

Diffuse damage includes:
- Diffuse axonal injury
- Hypoxic brain damage
- Diffuse brain swelling
- Diffuse vascular injury

Table 6.2   Initial management steps for patients with head injury

In the field
- Secure airway
- Administer O_2 by face mask
- Control bleeding
- Set up an infusion of i.v. fluids to maintain blood pressure
- Stabilize spine with cervical collar and back board
- During transport monitor blood pressure and O_2 saturation

In A & E
- Check and maintain a secure airway
- Intubate, paralyse and ventilate patients in coma
- Maintain $P_aCO_2 \approx 30–35\,mmHg$ and $P_aO_2 \approx 90\,mmHg$
- Treat shock
- Treat respiratory insufficiency
- Diagnose and stabilize extracranial injuries. Always obtain a CXR and arterial blood gases. **A lateral X-ray of the cervical spine to include T1 is essential to exclude injury.** Make sure the radiographer depresses the shoulders to avoid obscuring the T1 vertebra.
- Evaluate head injury

observation or to refer the patient to a neurosurgical unit. Criteria for admission are shown in Table 6.3. Discharged patients and their relative or carer should be issued with a Head Injury Warning Card (Fig. 6.1).

Keep the patient under observation. This should include monitoring the Glasgow Coma Score (GCS – Table 6.4) and assessment of blood pressure, pulse and O_2 saturation. Hypoxia is a common problem and there may not be obvious clinical signs – use pulse oximetry.

The **frequency of initial observations** is to a degree a matter of common sense. If the patient is fully conscious and there are no extracranial injuries, hourly observations are appropriate; once the patient is judged to be stable, the frequency of observations may be reduced to 4-hourly. If the patient is perceived to be at risk of an intracranial haematoma (e.g. fractured skull), continued hourly or half-hourly observations are likely to be required. If the patient has impairment of consciousness level (GCS 9–14), observations are required every 15–30 min. In severe head trauma, observations are required at least every 15 min. As the patient becomes more stable the frequency of observations may be reduced.

All patients in coma (GCS 8 or less) should have computed tomography (CT) as soon as possible after resuscitation. All patients in the categories listed in Table 6.5 will also require neurosurgical assessment or observation.

Keep all patients with a skull fracture in hospital for observation

Table 6.3   Criteria for admission of head-injured patients

- Depressed consciousness level
- Skull fracture
- Neurological symptoms/signs
- Difficult assessment
- No responsible carer

Southampton and South West Hampshire Health Authority

ACCIDENT AND EMERGENCY DEPARTMENT

NAME · THIS PERSON

HAS HAD AN INJURY TO THE HEAD ON ·
AND SHOULD RETURN TO HOSPITAL IMMEDIATELY OR
CONTACT YOUR OWN FAMILY DOCTOR IF THERE IS

> *DROWSINESS*
> *DIFFICULTY IN WAKING*
> *HEADACHE*
> *VOMITING*
> *FITS*

THIS PATIENT MUST NOT DRINK ALCOHOL

Fig. 6.1   Example of a head injury warning card.

Table 6.4   Glasgow Coma Scale

	Adults	*Children*	*Score*
Eye opening	Spontaneous	Spontaneous	4
	To speech	To sound	3
	To pain	To pain	2
	None	None	1
Verbal response	Orientated	Appropriate for age	5
	Confused	Cries	4
	Monosyllabic	Irritable	3
	Incomprehensible	Restless, lethargic	2
	None	None	1
Motor response	Obeys commands	Obeys commands (appropriate for age)	6
	Localizes to pain	Localizes to pain	5
	Flexion to pain	Flexion to pain	4
	Spastic flexion	Spastic flexion	3
	Extension to pain	Extension to pain	2
	None	None	1

Table 6.5   Criteria for CT scan and/or neurosurgical consultation

- Skull fracture with confusion
- Skull fracture with neurological signs
- Skull fracture and seizures
- GCS 9–14 after resuscitation
- Penetrating brain injury
- Depressed fracture

and ensure that the patient has a CT before discharge. Repeat the CT in any patient who remains drowsy for 24 hours. An early CT (within 6 hours) may have to be repeated to exclude a developing intracranial complication of head injury. If the repeat CT is normal, look for another cause for the patient's failure to improve.

Urgent transfer to the neurosurgical unit is required under the following circumstances:

- persisting coma after resuscitation;
- deterioration in consciousness level;
- open brain injury.

Examination of a head-injured patient

Consciousness level

Eye-opening, verbal response and motor responses are independently charted. An observation chart including these features is essential (see Table 6.4).

> This is the single most important assessment after the initial primary survey and is detailed using the GCS.

Pupil responses

The light reflex tests optic and oculomotor function. Oculomotor nerve function may be an adjunct in the detection of an expanding intracranial lesion. Herniation of the medial temporal lobe through the tentorial hiatus directly damages the third nerve, resulting in dilatation of the pupil with impaired or absent reaction to light.

> The pupil dilates on the side of the expanding lesion.

   Further increases in ICP may lead to bilateral fixed dilated pupils.

Eye movements

The presence or absence of abnormal eye movements is of limited value in immediate management issues but may have some prognostic significance. Abnormal eye movements are due to brain-stem dysfunction, damage to cranial nerves III–VI or vestibular damage. Absent eye movements are associated with a dismal prognosis.

   Cranial nerve damage is relatively uncommon. The nerves most often affected are II, VII and VIII. Assessing the cranial nerves fully in the unconscious patient is not possible. Signs to look for are shown in Table 6.6.

Limb weakness

This is determined by comparing the responses in each limb to a painful stimulus. Hemiparesis or hemiplegia usually occurs in the limbs contralateral to the side of the lesion. Limb responses are, however, of limited value as localizing signs because the ipsilateral limbs may be weak if there is indentation of the contralateral cerebral peduncle by the edge of the tentorium cerebelli.

> Early clinical assessment is invaluable as it predicts the requirement for further investigation and provides a baseline against which further changes can be compared. Make a careful and clear record of your findings and record the time of your examination.

   Essential features to record (present or absent/normal) are shown in Table 6.7.

Specific medical problems in head-injured patients

Cardiovascular

Hyperadrenergic activity and a hyperdynamic cardiovascular state will result in tachycardia, increased cardiac output, increased car-

Table 6.6 Signs commonly seen with cranial nerve injuries in head-injured patients

Cranial nerve	Aetiology	Clinical features	Outcome	Neurosurgical management
I	Anterior fossa fracture	Anosmia	Spontaneous resolution	No intervention
II	Fractures of the optic canal	Decreased acuity Reduced fields	Recovery unlikely	Optic nerve decompression
III, IV, VI	Fractures of the superior orbital fissure	Unequal pupils Deranged ocular movements	Spontaneous resolution	No intervention
V	Fractures of the petrous/sphenoid	Facial sensory loss	Recovery unlikely	No intervention
VII	Fractures of the petrous	Facial palsy	Recovery delayed in cases	Exploration/repair
IX, X, XI, XII (rare)	Fractures of the skull base	Cranial nerve palsies	Recovery unlikely	No intervention

Table 6.7 Examination of head-injured patients

Neurological
- Assess consciousness level (GCS)
- Pupils – size, symmetry and reactivity
- Cranial nerves
  - V
  - 'Doll's eyes'
  - Oculovestibular reflexes
  - Lower cranial nerves
- Eye movements
- Limb weakness
- External signs of trauma
- Signs of basal fracture such as CSF leak or bleeding from the nose or ear

Lacerations and bruising
- Explore scalp lacerations with gloved finger to feel for fractures

Features that suggest a basal skull fracture
- Anterior fossa
  - Bilateral periorbital swelling
  - Subconjunctival haematoma
  - CSF rhinorrhoea
- Middle fossa
  - CSF otorrhoea/bleeding
  - Bruising over mastoid
  - 'Battle's sign'

diac index and work, increased oxygen delivery and consumption, ECG abnormalities, myocardial ischaemia and pulmonary shunting. These require management in a neurosurgical intensive care (NITA) facility.

Metabolic

Head-injured patients are hypercatabolic, intolerant of glucose, may have fever and neutrophilia, readily lose total body protein and may have reduced levels of iron and zinc. Acute-phase proteins are readily detected and low transferrin, albumin and excessive nitrogen losses are associated with a poor neurological outcome. Nutritional needs must be addressed urgently with early total TPN until gastrointestinal function allows enteral nutrition.

Respiratory

Abnormal breathing patterns are common in severe head injury. This, in conjunction with the tendency towards dysfunctional pharyngeal reflexes, may lead to hypoxia. Ventilation/perfusion mismatches are common. Neurogenic pulmonary oedema may occur. This encompasses alveolar oedema, haemorrhage and congestion and is often associated with raised ICP. Adult respiratory distress syndrome (ARDS) may occur. Fat embolism may occur in severe polytrauma. Acute pulmonary embolism is a major contributor to morbidity and mortality and prophylaxis should be considered. These problems cannot be managed outside ITU/ NITA facilities.

Endocrine

Anterior and posterior pituitary dysfunction may occur. Hypothalamic dysfunction is common in severe head injury. In the acute phase management in a NITA facility is appropriate. Diabetes insipidus may occur in the acute or subacute phase. The diagnosis is confirmed by serum hypernatraemia and hyperosmolality; urine osmolality is low and sodium excretion is low. Diabetes insipidus is treated by administration of DDAVP. Do not start this treatment without neurosurgical consultation.

> Head-injured patients require careful i.v. fluid prescription and should never be dehydrated. Overhydration must also be avoided.

Gastric

Prophylactic gastric protection is justified to protect against the risk of GI bleeding. Gastroparesis and feeding intolerance may occur. Metoclopramide may improve gastric function. Parenteral nutrition may be required until gut function is normal.

Neurosurgical problems in the head-injured patient

Neurosurgical management of head-injured patients includes:

- operative and non-operative treatment of intracranial haematomas and contusions;
- management of raised intracranial pressure (ICP) and compromised CPP;
- prevention of intracranial infection;
- management of epilepsy;
- treatment of depressed fractures and penetrating brain injuries;
- craniofacial reconstruction after cranio-orbito-facial injury;
- management of CSF leaks.

Raised intracranial pressure

ICP depends on the volume of the intracranial contents. These include the brain, cerebrospinal fluid (CSF), cerebral blood volume (CBV) and the brain extracellular fluid (ECF).

CBV changes if cerebral blood flow (CBF) is altered. The brain receives 15% of the cardiac output; CBF is 800 ml/min. There is a close relationship between cerebral metabolism and CBF. CBF in turn is affected by arterial PaO_2, $PaCO_2$, systemic arterial blood pressure and temperature. Cerebral perfusion pressure (CPP) is the difference between mean systemic blood pressure (mABP) and ICP. Any increase in the volume of the skull contents leads to an increase in ICP. The relationship between pressure and volume is illustrated by the pressure–volume curve (Fig. 6.2).

Initially a rise in ICP is deferred by compensatory loss of CSF into the lumbar thecal sac or by a reduction in CBV. The slope of the pressure–volume curve depends on the rate of volume change. Eventually brain tissue is compressed, the brain shifts and herniation occurs and CBF falls, leading to global cerebral ischaemia. In the setting of an acute head injury, raised ICP may occur because of an expanding intracranial haematoma, brain swelling or cerebral oedema.

In the neurosurgical unit, raised ICP is controlled by evacuation of mass lesions; cerebral oedema, brain swelling and occult mass lesions are also treated using a combination of selective hyperventilation and the judicious use of mannitol or frusemide guided by intracranial pressure monitoring (mean ICP plus waveform analysis).

Outcome

In severe head injury recognized powerful independent predictors of outcome include:

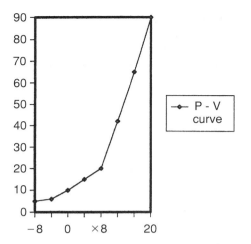

- ICP initially buffered by reduction CBV and displacement CSF into lumbar region
- subsequent decompensation and dramatic increase in ICP

Fig. 6.2 Pressure–volume curve. Intracranial pressure (ICP) is initially buffered by a reduction in cerebral blood volume and displacement of CSF into the lumbar region. Subsequent decompensation causes a dramatic increase in ICP.

- the GCS after resuscitation
- pupillary responses
- age
- ICP
- CT appearances.

After a severe head injury the overall mortality is about 36% for patients cared for in a dedicated NITA setting. In non-specialist units, mortality may be half as great again.

After minor or moderate head injury outcome varies widely depending on the nature of the head injury and associated extracranial injuries. A common problem after a minor head injury is the postconcussional syndrome. This is a self-limiting disorder of memory and concentration, with persisting headache. No specific treatment is required.

Summary

Head injury is complex. The basics are simple. Significant morbidity and mortality can be avoided by attention to detail.

- Avoid hypoxia.
- Avoid hypotension – the biggest enemy of the head-injured patient.

Complications remote from the head are similar to those seen in patients with burns or multiple trauma. In patients with a severe head injury or a moderately severe head injury complicated by extracranial injuries the lowest morbidity and mortality rates occur when there is awareness of the potential problems that threaten brain recovery and when the patient is nursed in an intensive care or NITA facility.

SURGERY FOR HEAD INJURY

Intracranial haematoma

Craniotomy is now the mainstay of surgery for all traumatic intracranial haematoma whether extradural, subdural or intracerebral. The days of exploratory (educated guesswork) burr holes are gone; 'tailor-made' flaps over the haematoma as demonstrated by CT are now routine. Apart from exceptional circumstances, operations should not be done outside a neurosurgical unit; better primary management, early diagnosis, safe interhospital transfer and lower admission thresholds by neurosurgeons have all played their part in transferring patients promptly to centres with the appropriate clinical experience.

The indications for surgery are usually fairly clear, with some room for clinical judgement. A moderate to large haematoma with mass effect and clinical deterioration is an absolute indication for operation provided the patient is neither unstable from the cardiorespiratory point of view nor *in extremis* (neurologically or otherwise) such that treatment would be fruitless. Small haematomas also occur and here only experience dictates the value or otherwise of removal – the decision is based upon a number of factors including the age, the neurological state (GCS) and the nature and severity of other injuries.

Anaesthesia

High-quality anaesthetic support is critical to the management of head injury. There is no place for the 'amateur intubator', as poor technique readily causes raised intracranial pressure. Coughing, gagging, struggling, raised $P_a\mathrm{co}_2$ and reduced $P_a\mathrm{co}_2$ all increase intracranial pressure, with the obvious implications for intubation, maintenance of anaesthesia and mechanical ventilation. The head-injured patient is also at risk of obstructed/damaged airway, chest injury and altered central control of respiration. However, competent anaesthesia can have considerable therapeutic benefit, not least by correcting abnormal blood gases. Hyperventilation is equally valuable in the short term and, in lowering $P_{\#a}\backslash scco\backslash rt_{\#2}$, also lowers intracranial pressure. Unfortunately, this effect is usually lost after about 24 hours, but it can buy valuable time in the acute situation. Also of value in acutely lowering intracranial pressure is the intravenous administration of 20% mannitol. Unfortunately, this cannot be given regularly as it leaks into the tissues and can then have the reverse osmotic effect of encouraging cerebral oedema. Its use, therefore, is limited to being an adjunct to surgery and situations of significantly raised intracranial pressure where there is no other alternative.

The operation – craniotomy

Plan the incision carefully.

Head position

Position the patient slightly head-up (to reduce intracranial venous pressure) with the flap uppermost. If the dura is opened, this stops the brain from prolapsing under gravity and helps considerably with closure of the dura.

The flap

The flap should be broad-based (to ensure good vascular supply). Do not make the incision over the forehead (for cosmetic reasons). Always check you are operating on the correct side of the head; this seems obvious but in the heat of the moment mistakes can happen. Check and double-check the CT. Remember that modern scanners look at the brain as if from below; hence the left side of the brain is on the right side of the scan picture.

Although the flap should be placed over the haematoma there are two standard skin flaps that are commonly used, as most haematomas are centred on or around the pterion (Fig. 6.3).

The scalp is very vascular and it is helpful to infiltrate the skin and not the subgaleal plane (which is much easier to do) with a solution of local anaesthetic and adrenaline (check with the anaesthetist the permitted dose). Incise the skin through the galea but try not to cut the underlying periosteum (you need that to suture the bone flap back in at the end). Once the galea is cut, the skin edges pull apart easily. Incise the skin in short sections (approximately 10 cm) and, after each cut, place haemostats on the cut edges – usually specially designed plastic clips, although artery forceps are equally effective.

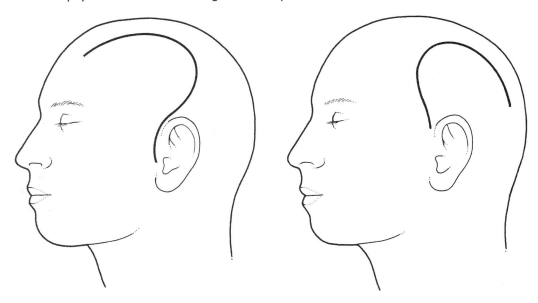

Fig. 6.3   Standard skin flaps used for haematoma.

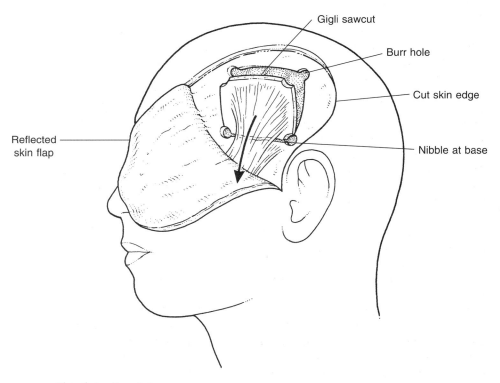

Fig. 6.4   Craniotomy.

Make the bone flap using either a craniotome or four burr holes and gently separate the dura from the undersurface of the bone with a blunt dissector. Make intervening saw cuts on three sides (but not the base – see Fig. 6.4) with a Gigli saw. Then 'nibble' a small amount of bone on both sides of the base of the flap, under the muscle, to make it easier to crack the bone at this point.

An extradural haematoma strips the dura away from the bone but in all other cases you must strip the dura manually before elevating the bone flap. It is easier to get the blunt dissector under the bone if the flap is gently levered up a few millimetres. Remember, the older the patient, the more adherent the dura is to the bone.

Once you have made all the saw cuts, nibbled the base and separated the dura, lever up the bone flap and fracture it across the base (Fig. 6.4).

Thus far the procedure is the same for acute extra- and subdural haematoma but thereafter the technique is quite different.

> When elevating the bone flap be mindful of the position of any skull fracture, as the flap may crack across the fracture rather than where you intended.

Extradural haematoma   Once the bone flap is elevated, remove the haematoma by suction to expose the dura. If necessary, gently elevate the clot with a blunt dissector. Remember, the dura only provides limited protection to the underlying brain, which is very delicate.

Ignore the folklore that surrounds stemming the bleeding from the middle meningeal artery (matchsticks in foramen spinosum, etc.). First, it is often not bleeding by this stage of the operation and if it is, it can be easily controlled with bipolar diathermy. Do not 'fry' the dura excessively (it often oozes a bit) because it shrinks when diathermied and this tents it away from the undersurface of the bone and makes it very difficult at the end to obliterate the extradural space by 'hitching' the dura to the pericranium (see below). Sometimes there is brisk haemorrhage from deep in the temporal fossa. Avoid long and fruitless efforts to control this with diathermy; it can usually be stopped with a combination of haemostatic gauze, hitching of the dura and patience.

Acute subdural haematoma   The position of these varies little and most are centred in or around the pterion; hence one of the two flaps described above usually suffices.

The major challenge of acute subdural haematomas is that they usually overlie a swollen, injured brain and once the dura is opened, not only does the haematoma frequently 'express' itself but the brain may also 'mushroom' alarmingly through the defect. This is not only very damaging to the herniating brain but can also make closure extremely difficult. To avoid this, do not open the dura widely (tempting though it may be): open the dura through small 2–3 cm incisions

If the patient is deteriorating quickly, an extradural haematoma can be rapidly decompressed in a few minutes using a sucker through the first burr hole before you raise the flap. Similarly, decompress an acute subdural haematoma by opening the dura through the most appropriate burr hole, but remember that immediately below the clot is the brain, which is friable at the best of times but even more so after trauma.

over the haematoma and hold the edges gently apart. The clot frequently extrudes itself but gentle suction and encouragement with a blunt dissector may be necessary. This technique, methodically performed, produces a perfectly adequate decompression. Wide opening of the dura can be performed if the brain is slack, but beware: it can occasionally swell very rapidly – this procedure is best left to an experienced neurosurgeon.

Closure

Hitching the dura to the pericranium (or temporalis muscle) is important to obliterate the extradural space and prevent a postoperative extradural haematoma. Some also add a central suture passed through a hole in the bone flap. This is a fiddly business as it is imperative not to go through the dura and catch a cerebral cortical vessel, which will result in a postoperative subdural haematoma. Use a fine suture needle and pick up the dura with fine-toothed forceps.

Haemostasis

Meticulous haemostasis is essential as postoperative intracranial haematoma is a potentially fatal complication. Hitching the dura reduces bleeding from under the bone edges and bleeding from the dura itself can be controlled by bipolar diathermy. Control bleeding from the bone with bone wax.

Bone

Return the bone flap and suture it to the pericranium and muscle (usually temporalis).

Wound drainage and skin closure

Place a closed suction drain in the subgaleal space and maintain low-pressure suction for 24–48 hours. Do not use the high suction pressures used in other branches of surgery, which can have devastating effects, presumably through negative intracranial pressure.

Skin

Close the skin in two layers with an absorbable (2/0) suture in the galea aponeurotica – this can be either continuous or interrupted. Skin closure is standard but staples, are quick, easy and effective.

Intracranial pressure monitoring

This can be performed in conjunction with craniotomy for haematoma, or as a primary procedure where there is no surgical lesion but the suggestion of raised intracranial pressure (ICP) on the CT.

ICP can be measured from the lateral ventricles, the subdural space, the brain parenchyma or extradural space. The latter is the least invasive but the least accurate. Measurement from the lateral ventricles is invasive and the benefit of being able to withdraw cerebrospinal fluid to relieve high ICP is quickly lost as the ventricular walls collapse. New techniques are available to measure pressure from the parenchyma but these are not yet widely used and require expensive special equipment. Subdural pressure monitoring is a good compromise, is less invasive and is pretty reliable.

The risks of this technique are almost exclusively related to infection, as the measuring catheter has to be brought out through the skin. Haematoma formation is rare.

Operative technique

As a primary procedure, insert the monitor through a standard burr hole – usually frontal. Site the frontal burr hole approximately 5 cm behind the hairline and 3 cm from the midline (make burr holes over the midline at your peril: remember the position of the venous sinuses). Infiltrate the skin as described above and make a 5–6 cm 'paramedian' incision straight down to the bone; scrape the pericranium to either side with a blunt dissector and insert a self-retaining retractor, which usually stems any bleeding from the skin.

Use the time-honoured Hudson brace to make a standard burr hole – as the inner table is breached, the feel of the perforator goes from being relatively smooth to feeling like a ratchet. Take care to control the perforator as it is all too easy to 'plunge' into the brain. Once the feeling changes, stop – you should be able to see a small central hole through which the dura can be felt with the tips of a pair of forceps. Then change to the 'burr' to complete the hole.

Next, open the dura using a small sharp hook and fine blade. Cut a cruciate incision in the dura with fine scissors and diathermy the edges to stop any bleeding. This will also cause them to retract. For insertion of a subdural pressure monitor, tunnel a standard ventricular catheter about 4–5 cm through the skin. Gently retract the brain surface away and slide the wet proximal end into the subdural space a distance of at least 6 cm. This procedure requires great care, and the higher the ICP, the more difficult it is. While the wound is open, connect the catheter to a three-way tap and prime the tubing with sterile saline for injection, allowing any excess to drain from the subdural space. Avoid air bubbles in the line, as these cause inaccurate pressure recording.

Closure is simple: put three or four interrupted absorbable sutures in the galea and then use a standard skin closure.

Otolaryngology

Christopher J. Randall

7

TRACHEOSTOMY

Definition

Tracheostomy is the creation of a direct passage into the trachea, bypassing the upper airway.

Indications

Actual or anticipated upper airway obstruction, or for direct access to the airway for suction or long-term ventilation.
   Generally this falls into three categories:

- urgent relief of airway obstruction caused by facial trauma, laryngeal infection or tumour;
- prophylactic protection of the airway in operations around the upper airway, e.g. head and neck cancer operations, some cases of anterior spinal fusion and operations on the larynx;
- for long-term ventilatory support on intensive care units or in chronic airways disease.

> If you are in doubt as to whether to do a tracheostomy – **do one.**

Anaesthesia

Local anaesthesia may often be the safest in the acute situation. Position the patient half sitting up and infiltrate the skin and deeper tissues with copious 0.5% lignocaine. Inject further local anaesthetic throughout the procedure if required.
   When general anaesthesia is contemplated the closest cooperation is required between the anaesthetist and surgeon. Induction should be with gaseous anaesthesia. Avoid intravenous agents and paralysis, which may precipitate complete obstruction with disastrous consequences. In the emergency situation a tracheostomy set should be opened and ready in the anaesthetic room in case the airway is lost during induction and subsequent intubation then proves impossible.

Incision

Extend the neck by a pad under the shoulders. Make a skin-crease transverse incision midway between the cricoid and the suprasternal notch. Extend it laterally to the anterior borders of sterno-cleidomastoid. A small incision gives no better scar, but makes the procedure much harder and more hazardous.

The operation

Deepen the incision down to the strap muscles, dividing and tying the anterior jugular veins on the way. Separate the first layer of strap muscles (sternohyoids) in the midline and retract them laterally. Next separate the thinner sternothyroid muscles in the midline and partially lift them off the thyroid gland to reveal the thyroid isthmus.

Divide and transfix the thyroid isthmus to reveal the anterior wall of the trachea. In adults remove the anterior part of a tracheal ring. Never excise the first tracheal ring as damage to this can lead to late tracheal stenosis. The second, third or fourth ring is suitable (Fig. 7.1).

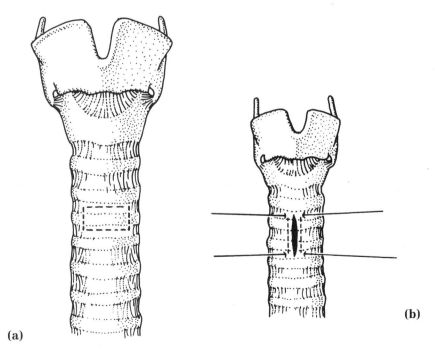

(a)

(b)

Fig. 7.1 Position of incision in the trachea. **(a)** Adult. **(b)** Child.

Before you enter the trachea, allow the anaesthetist to free the endotracheal tube and check yourself all tubes and connections. Only then may you remove the anterior tracheal ring, withdraw the endotracheal tube and insert the tracheostomy tube directly into the trachea. Finally, the cuff is inflated and the tube is connected to the anaesthetic machine.

Closure

Tie the tube securely in place. Do not tie it too tightly and close the skin very loosely. An airtight closure may lead to surgical emphysema.

Postoperative care

The inspired air should be kept humidified for the first few days and the tube should be sucked out initially 2-hourly. The frequency of suction can be reduced according to need.

Crash tracheostomy

In the life-saving acute situation, tracheostomy is performed mostly by feel. Make a vertical incision and deepen the incision between fingers that feel their way down to the trachea. Make a vertical incision in the tracheal wall and insert the tube. You then have time to achieve haemostasis at leisure.

Tracheostomy in children

In children various modifications must be made to the standard operation. First the entry into the trachea must be a vertical slit, not the removal of a ring. Second, as the tube is more likely to come out and can be very difficult to replace, place stay sutures in the trachea on either side of the vertical slit before inserting the tube. Bring these out to the skin and tape them down. If the tube falls out, gentle traction on these sutures should show the way back in. They can be removed after the first tube change, 5 days to a week after operation.

Changing the tube

The first tube change can take place after 3–4 days when the track has stabilized. Have at hand a sucker with both Yankauer and catheter ends, tracheal dilators and tracheostomy tubes of the same size and one size smaller.

The tracheostomy hole is largest on expiration. Instruct the patient to take a deep breath in and hold his/her breath. Remove the old tube and insert the new one following the curve of the track into the trachea. Tapes should be loose enough to fit four fingers easily between tape and neck.

Removal of the tube

Before a tracheostomy tube is removed, carry out a trial with the tube blocked. Place an uncuffed tracheostomy tube so adequate ventilation is possible around the tube. Cork the tube for 24 hours. If there is no distress the tube can simply be taken out. Cover the hole with an airtight bandage and it will close rapidly and spontaneously.

PACKING A NOSE

Preparations

Anaesthetize the nose by spraying in either lignocaine or cocaine 10%. If the blood flow is considerable, pack the nose loosely. Use a pack soaked in cocaine 5% or lignocaine and then wrung out.

Packing

If you anticipate that the pack will be *in situ* for more than 24 hours then it should be impregnated with bismuth paraffin paste (BIPP). Failure to do this will result in a foul pack and a risk of secondary haemorrhage. First insert a nasal speculum into the nose, then pack loops of ribbon along the floor of the nose. Pack down each loop with a sucker before you introduce the next loop above it and pack it down in turn. In this fashion a tight pack can be reliably inserted to tamponade any bleeding (Fig. 7.2).

Inserting a postnasal pack

Indications

If bleeding continues down the nasopharynx despite a good anterior nasal pack.

Making the pack

Make the pack by folding a tonsil swab into three and then folding another one on top of this. Sew the whole pack together with through and through silk stitches. Sew a ribbon on to each side half way along

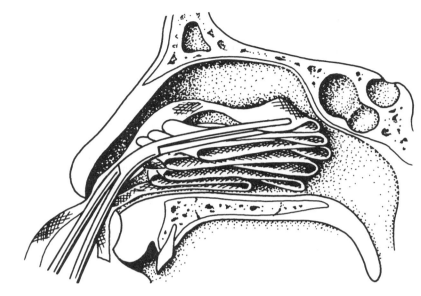

Fig. 7.2   Insertion of an anterior nasal pack.

its length to make an elongated H with the pack as the cross bar. Soak the whole pack in BIPP (Fig. 7.3).

Insertion

Insert a postnasal pack under general anaesthesia. Remove the anterior pack and insert a Boyle–Davis gag into the mouth to hold open the jaw. Pass a Jaques catheter through each nostril and out through the mouth. Tie one end of each ribbon to each catheter. Draw the catheters back through the nose to take the postnasal pack into the nasopharynx. Free the catheters from the ribbons and tie them over a dental swab under the columella (midline) of the nose. Do not leave this too tight or uncushioned as it will cause necrosis of the columella and lead to serious deformity.

Tape the other end of the ribbons loosely to the cheek; they will be used later for removal of the pack. Finally replace the anterior nasal pack (Fig. 7.4).

Removal of a postnasal pack

On the ward cut the ribbons tied under the anterior nose and remove the knot. Free the tapes on the cheek, insert a finger along one of these to the back of the mouth, and then flick the pack down from the nasopharynx and withdraw it.

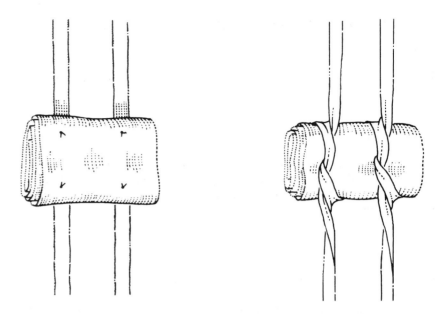

Fig. 7.3 Preparation of a postnasal pack.

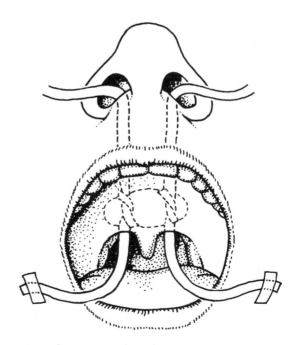

Fig. 7.4 Insertion of a postnasal pack.

DIRECT LARYNGOSCOPY AND PHARYNGOSCOPY

Definition

Examination of the larynx and pharynx with rigid instruments under anaesthesia.

Indications

Inability to examine the larynx properly by indirect or fibreoptic methods, or the need to take a biopsy. The pharynx, and in particular the hypopharynx, can only be adequately examined by rigid instruments.

Important points

- Warn the patient of possible damage to the teeth and take great care to protect them throughout the procedure.
- The examination of the larynx is bimanual. Once the laryngoscope is down at the larynx, move the larynx around the instrument to visualize all areas.
- It is important to be totally systematic about examining all areas and record carefully all the results in the various sites. In order to maintain this discipline it is a good idea to write down after each operation the results in the following area checklist:
  - Tongue
  - Vallecula
  - Aryepiglottic folds
  - False cords
  - Laryngeal ventricle
  - Cords
  - Subglottis
  - Pyriform fossa
  - Cricothyroid area.

Anaesthesia

The surgeon and anaesthetist are trying to share the same airway. Many methods have been devised to get round this problem, but in my view one can usually obtain an adequate view round a small (5–6 mm) cuffed endotracheal tube. This is safe and simple. Generally the examination is easier and less traumatic if the patient is paralysed.

Positioning

The correct position is with the neck flexed and the head extended. This is achieved by putting a pillow under the head but not the shoulder.

Examination

Place a tooth guard over the teeth; in the edentulous patient place a wet swab on the upper gum. Rest the left index or middle finger on the upper teeth and push open the lower jaw with the thumb. As you insert the laryngoscope into the gap move your left thumb off the lower teeth to take up position behind the scope, preventing it from levering directly on the upper teeth. In this way, manoeuvre the endoscope to look at all parts of the larynx. At completion of the examination, withdraw the laryngoscope. Insert the longer pharyngoscope in the same fashion to view the pyriform fossae and postcricoid area. Lastly, palpate the base of the tongue with a finger.

Postoperatively

If there has been any trauma in the lower pharynx, examine the patient 2–3 hours postoperatively to enquire about any pain and to check for surgical emphysema of the neck. Obtain a lateral X-ray of the neck to check for signs of free gas.

NASAL POLYPECTOMY

Important points

- Polypectomy is an operation to cure symptoms and not to extirpate disease. Therefore you do not need to be unduly radical.
- Every year people lose their vision or develop CSF leaks as a result of excessive zeal when landmarks are lost. Do not get carried away.
- Unilateral polyps may be malignant so must always be sent for histology.

Anatomical points

Do not go medial to or above the middle turbinate as this leads to the cribriform plate. The lateral wall of the ethmoidal complex is the lamina papyracea, which is very thin. Do not go to far laterally. Throughout the procedure watch the eye carefully. To facilitate this the lids should not be taped shut.

Under local anaesthesia

Polypectomy can be very adequately performed in many situations under local anaesthesia. Wrap cotton wool on a silver probe and dip it in cocaine 25% paste. If there are medical contraindications to cocaine then use lignocaine 5% instead. Paint the nasal cavity with the solution and leave the probe far back under the middle turbinate for at least 15 min. Sit the patient up in a dental chair and instruct him/her to spit out anything that falls backwards into the mouth.

It is important not to pull if pain is to be avoided. Use a cutting snare. Each polyp is lassooed from medial to lateral, cut and then removed with a sucker. Properly performed, the procedure should be virtually painless and blood-free (Fig. 7.5).

General anaesthesia

General anaesthesia is performed with appropriate protection of the airway. Place the patient supine on a head ring and paint the nasal cavity with cocaine 25% paste. It is possible to be more radical under general anaesthesia. Grasp the polyps in forceps and push backwards to avulse the stalk, and then pull the polyp out of the nose. Take care to remain lateral to and beneath the middle turbinate. The turbinate itself should be left carefully intact as a landmark.

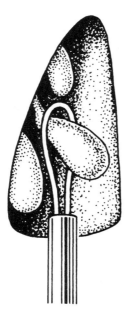

Fig. 7.5 Snaring of a polyp.

Packing

If there is significant bleeding at the end of the operation the nose should be packed. Generally, this can be a light pack of paraffin ribbon, which can be removed the next morning.

TONSILLECTOMY

Indications

- Recurrent acute tonsillitis not controlled by conservative treatment;
- Upper airway obstruction from large tonsils and adenoids;
- Histological analysis;
- Access to deeper structures such as the styloid process.

Anaesthesia

Use general anaesthesia with an endotracheal tube to safeguard the airway. This is usually an oral tube carefully fixed in the midline. In adults, some surgeons favour a nasotracheal tube.

Position

Place the patient supine with a pad under the shoulder to extend the neck and a small head ring to steady the head. Apply soft paraffin to the corner of the mouth to prevent trauma from instruments.

Operation

The secret of tonsillectomy is to grasp and free the upper pole; the rest of the dissection is then fairly straightforward.

Insert a Boyle–Davis gag and open it, taking care to keep the tongue in the midline. Suspend the gag with Draffins rods to leave both your hands free.

Initially, grasp the upper pole of the tonsil with Luc's or Denis Browne forceps, and pull it medially. It is important that this grasping of the tonsil should be as high up as it is possible to place the forceps cups. Incise the mucosa along the anterior pillar and up over the superior pole, freeing the uvula. Continue the incision down the posterior pillar. Still grasping the superior pole, free the capsule off the superior pole with a dissector, allowing the grip of the forceps to be changed to one blade medial and one lateral to the lower pole. Thus grasped, draw the tonsil medially and continue with blunt dissection behind the tonsil to the lower pole. At this stage, pass a snare carefully over the tonsil and shave off the final attachment at the lower pole. Pack the tonsil bed with a tonsil swab. Remove the other tonsil in the same way (Fig. 7.6).

Leave the packs in place for a few minutes and most of the bleeding will stop. Remaining vessels can then be stopped by ties and/or diathermy. Do not perform tonsillectomy until you can tie single-handed knots and tighten them over forceps with either hand.

Single-handed knots First grasp the bleeding vessel in straight Burkett's forceps, and then pass semicurved Negus forceps under the vessel, and remove the Burkett's. Wind a linen tie round the ring finger of the hand opposite the tonsil being tied, in order to anchor the end. Hold a pusher between the index finger and thumb of the same hand and bowstring the tie over the pusher while you hold the other end in the hand on the same side as the tonsil. Pass a single-handed throw down the string and tighten it with the pusher. At the same time ask your assistant to release and remove the Negus forceps. Repeat this to place further throws to secure the ligature. When the tonsil bed is dry remove the gag, close the jaw and make sure that the patient is extubated in the supine position with the head down.

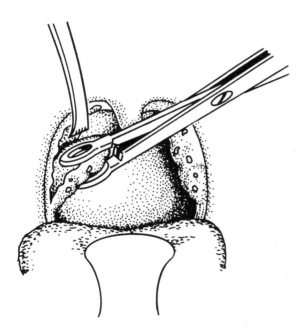

Fig. 7.6 Dissection of the tonsil from the tonsillar fossa.

Postoperative care

The major risk in tonsillectomy is that the airway may become blocked by blood clot before a vigorous cough reflex has returned. Make sure the patient is monitored carefully during recovery from anaesthesia and avoid opiate analgesics. In children, use rectal diclofenac and insert the suppository while the child is still asleep. In both children and adults, avoid aspirin in view of its effect on platelet function. Diclofenac, ibuprofen and paracetamol are usually all that is required. Eating of solid food is encouraged as soon as postoperative nausea has passed.

ADENOIDECTOMY

Indications

- Acute or serious otitis media;
- Recurrent upper respiratory tract bacterial infections;
- Nasal obstruction, especially in sleep apnoea.

Anaesthesia

General anaesthesia with an oral endotracheal tube.

Position

Place the patient supine with a head ring but not a sandbag. If adenoidectomy is performed at the same time as tonsillectomy, the head should be flexed and lifted slightly to offset the effect of the sandbag.

Operation

Pass an adenoid curette behind the palate and back until it abuts on to the back of the nasal septum. Taking care to keep the handle of the curette vertical, drive the curette downwards towards the operating table and into the adenoid pad. Then rotate it forward in an arc round the upper incisors, protecting them with the thumb of your other hand. In this way you can sweep the adenoid into the oropharynx and remove it. Repeat the same procedure at either side with a small unguarded curette, again keeping the handle strictly vertical to avoid damaging the eustachian cushions.

Palpate the nasopharynx with a finger to check there is no remaining adenoid tissue before you insert a pack with tonsil swabs. After about 2 min remove the swabs and generally the bleeding will have

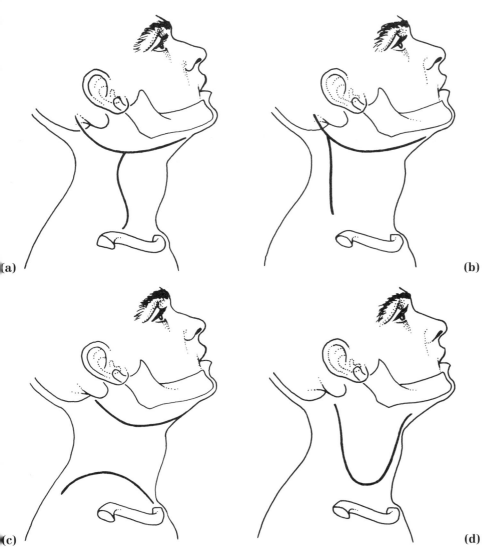

Fig. 7.7 Incisions for a neck dissection. **(a)** Y-incision. **(b)** Modified Schobinger. **(c)** Modified McFee; **(d)** Apron.

stopped. If it fails to stop, replace the packing until it does. In the unusual event of persistent bleeding insert a postnasal pack.

Recovery

The patient is recovered in the 'tonsillar' position. Generally only simple analgesia is required.

ASSESSMENT OF NECK LYMPH NODE

No lymph node should ever be removed for biopsy until a detailed attempt has been made to discover its nature and ascertain whether there is a primary tumour in the head and neck. Failure to do this may seriously reduce your patient's ultimate prognosis.

Step 1

Take a fine needle aspiration of the lump. The technique is the same as for any other lump (Chapter 1). Squamous cell carcinoma is generally easy to diagnose by this method. If this is found, the primary is almost certainly in the head and neck and must then be sought for. Lymphomas are more difficult, but an experienced pathologist usually picks up the malignant nature of the lymphocytes. More importantly, squamous cell carcinoma and lymphoma are unlikely to be confused.

Step 2

Make a thorough search for the primary. Search the skin carefully, then inspect the mouth, tongue, nasopharynx, pharynx, larynx and hypopharynx (under anaesthesia if necessary) and obtain a chest X-ray. The most likely primary sites to be missed are the nasopharynx, posterior third of tongue, tonsil and pyriform fossa. If fine-needle aspiration shows squamous cell carcinoma and there is no obvious primary site, then take random biopsies of these sites ipsilaterally.

Step 3

Only if no primary is found after a thorough search the node should be biopsied. If fine-needle aspiration shows squamous cell carcinoma then there is a strong case for performing a radical neck dissection rather than a node biopsy. If you are asked to perform a node biopsy, site the incision so that it can be incorporated in a subsequent neck dissection if that proves necessary (Fig. 7.7).

Ophthalmology

8

Louise E. Allen

Eye disease may be encountered both in the Accident and Emergency Department and on the surgical ward. While a specialized knowledge of ophthalmology is not expected of a basic surgical trainee, you should be able to perform a competent eye examination, initiate emergency eye care and treat the more common ocular complaints. This chapter outlines these essential skills.

BASIC EYE EXAMINATION

The tools required for a basic eye examination are:

- Pen-torch
- Snellen chart
- Ophthalmoscope
- Fluorescein 1% or 2% drops or fluorescein paper strips
- Topical anaesthetic drops: oxybuprocaine 0.4% or amethocaine 1%
- Mydriatic drops: tropicamide 1%.

Although the following paragraphs provide a framework for an eye assessment, you should tailor the ophthalmic examination to the patient's circumstances and omit any inappropriate steps.

Examination of the orbit

Inspect the lids, documenting your findings with diagrams. Compare the prominence of the globes by standing behind the seated patient and looking downwards over the brow. Proptosis or enophthalmos may cause one eye to look more prominent than the other. If you suspect an orbital floor fracture, feel for discontinuity along the orbital rim, palpate the surrounding skin for surgical emphysema and test for hypoaesthesia over the lower lid and cheek. In cases where ocular infection may be present, palpate the preauricular lymph nodes for enlargement and tenderness.

Examination of eye movements

Using a pen-torch as a target for visual pursuit, slowly move the torch so that it describes an H pattern centred at the patient's primary position of gaze. This will enable you to assess the function of each extraocular muscle in turn (Fig. 8.1).

The corneal light reflection in each eye will disappear if you move the torch beyond the range of eye movement or if the view from the eye becomes occluded, e.g. by the bridge of the nose. Document the eye position in which the patient reports diplopia and whether the diplopia is monocular, binocular, vertical or horizontal in nature. Express the range of ocular motility in each direction as a percentage of normal.

Measurement of visual acuity

If the patient is in pain, instil a few drops of topical anaesthetic prior to measurement. With the patient wearing their distance glasses (if available) and standing 6 metres from a Snellen chart, grade the visual acuity from 6/4 to 6/60. If the largest letter cannot be read, halve the distance from the chart (the numerator now being 3, e.g. 3/60). For patients with poorer vision, assess the ability to count fingers (CF), appreciate hand movement (HM) or perceive light (PL). Improvement in acuity when the chart is viewed through a pinhole suggests a refractive error.

Examination of the visual fields

The visual field of each eye should be tested. If the field loss is unilateral, the contours of the defect should help localize the prob-

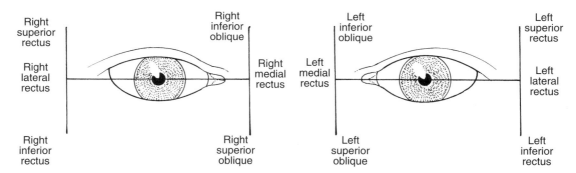

Ocular (third) nerve innervates: levator palpebre superioris, superior, inferior and medial recti muscle inferior oblique muscle
Trochlear (fourth) nerve innervates: superior oblique muscle
Abducent (sixth) nerve innervates: lateral rectus muscle

Fig. 8.1 The muscles controlling eye movements and their innervation.

lem: a central scotoma results from optic nerve or macular pathology; an altitudinal field defect (loss of the superior or inferior half of the visual field) from vascular occlusion. Retinal detachment causes an enlarging peripheral field defect, which eventually interferes with central vision. Bilateral field loss (e.g. homonymous hemianopia) usually implies an extraocular cause.

Examination of pupillary reactions

Test the pupillary reactions in a darkened room with the patient looking into the distance. Compare pupillary size, then examine the direct and consensual light response. A defect in the **efferent** pupillary pathway (e.g. oculomotor (third) nerve palsy or traumatic mydriasis) prevents pupillary constriction, resulting in a larger, non-reacting pupil, although the other will react normally to both direct and consensual stimuli. A defect in the **afferent** pupillary pathway (i.e. from retina to optic tract) may be complete or partial. A **complete afferent pupillary defect** prevents light perception by that eye; the pupils are equal because both eyes respond to the light sensed by the normal eye, but if a light is shone in the blind eye neither pupil reacts. A partial or **relative afferent pupillary defect** (RAPD) causes the light in the defective eye to be sensed as 'less bright' than when appreciated by the normal eye, so although a small direct and consensual light reaction occurs, this is less than that resulting from stimulation of the normal eye. This may be demonstrated by the swinging torch test: as the light approaches the normal eye, both pupils constrict; as the torch is swung to the abnormal eye, the pupils dilate slightly. It is important to test for an RAPD since a positive response indicates serious ocular and optic nerve pathology which might otherwise remain undetected.

Red desaturation (reduced sensitivity to the colour red) is another important sign of optic nerve pathology. Ask the patient to compare the brightness of a red target shown to each eye in turn: the target will appear 'washed out' or darker when viewed by the affected eye.

Examination of the anterior segment

If the patient is in pain, instil topical anaesthetic to facilitate examination. Gently retract the lower lid and examine the inferior conjunctival fornix. Evert the upper lid to expose the superior subtarsal conjunctiva as shown in Fig. 8.2.

Examine the cornea with a pen-torch; a magnified image can be achieved by viewing the cornea through an ophthalmoscope set on +20 dioptres. Instil either a drop of fluorescein or a fluorescein paper strip moistened with topical anaesthetic into the inferior fornix. An

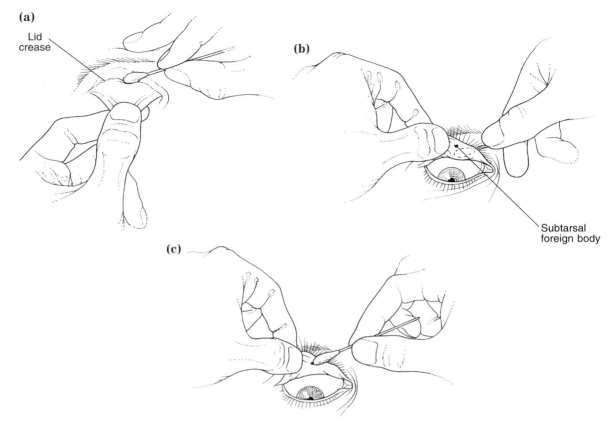

(a)

Lid crease

(b)

Subtarsal foreign body

(c)

Fig. 8.2 Method of everting the upper eyelid. **(a)** Place the tip of the cotton bud on to the lid crease. While pushing towards the globe, grasp the upper eyelashes and pivot the lid around the cotton bud. **(b)** Inspect the subtarsal region for a foreign body. **(c)** Remove the foreign body using a moistened cotton bud.

area of conjunctival or corneal epithelial loss will fluoresce yellow-green under blue light (most ophthalmoscopes are fitted with a blue filter). Describe the position of any pathology using clock hours of the cornea's circumference. Assess the depth of the anterior chamber by shining the torch obliquely across the cornea: the quadrant of iris furthest away from the torch will be illuminated by the beam if the anterior chamber is of normal depth, but if the chamber is shallow the iris will bow forwards and the far quadrant will remain in shadow.

Fundoscopy

The risk of precipitating angle-closure glaucoma by pharmacological mydriasis is slight and should not preclude dilated fundoscopy when it is indicated. However, warn patients over 45 years of age to return if eye ache, nausea or visual haloes occur. Tropicamide acts in 20 min and lasts for 3 hours, during which time the patient should not drive a motor vehicle. Compare the quality of the red reflex in both eyes and note the colour, cup and margin of the optic disc. Examine the macula by asking the patient to look towards the light of the ophthalmoscope.

APPEARANCES AFTER COMMON EYE OPERATIONS

Intraocular surgery can alter the appearance of the eye and awareness of the common operations may prevent some embarrassing referrals.

Cataract surgery

Intracapsular cataract extraction

The lens nucleus and capsule are removed, leaving the patient either without a lens (aphakic) or with a prosthetic intraocular lens (IOL) positioned anterior to the iris, where it is visible on pen-torch examination (Fig. 8.3).

Extracapsular cataract extraction and IOL

In this more common technique, the lens nucleus only is removed, leaving the capsule *in situ* to support the IOL behind the iris, where

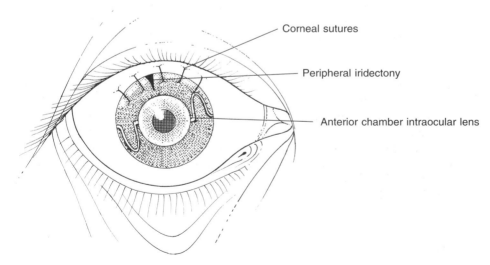

Corneal sutures

Peripheral iridectony

Anterior chamber intraocular lens

Fig. 8.3 The appearance of an eye after cataract extraction with an anterior chamber intraocular lens.

it is invisible on pen-torch examination. Sutures are present from 10 to 2 o'clock along the superior corneal limbus. These may break many months after surgery, giving a foreign body sensation and requiring removal. If the cataract is phacoemulsified and aspirated within the capsular bag rather than expressed from the eye, a smaller incision is made, which does not require sutures.

Glaucoma surgery

A trabeculectomy is commonly performed for chronic open-angle glaucoma. A communication is made between the anterior chamber and the subconjunctival space, where aqueous humour is slowly absorbed. A conjunctival bleb at the superior limbus and a triangular defect in the iris (peripheral iridectomy) may be visible.

COMMON EYE THERAPY

Many ocular medications are available in both drop (*guttae – g.*) or ointment (*oculentum – oc.*) form. The form prescribed depends on the patient's circumstances; ointments lubricate and ease pain but blur vision, making them less suitable for bilateral conditions. If you are unsure of the diagnosis or correct therapy, seek advice from an ophthalmologist before starting treatment. Topical steroid and ocular hypotensive therapy should not be initiated by a non-specialist.

Antibiotics

Oc. chloramphenicol 1%, *g.* chloramphenicol 0.5% or *g.* fusidic acid 1% are suitable for antibacterial prophylaxis after minor trauma and mild ocular infections.

Treatment of allergy

Mast cell stabilizers such as *g.* sodium cromoglycate 2% or *g.* lodoxamide may be used throughout the hay-fever season. Antihistamines, e.g. *g.* antazoline, control severe itching following exposure to the allergen.

Analgesics

Topical anaesthesic agents delay epithelial healing and have no therapeutic role. Treatments for specific conditions are described later.

Ocular lubricants

Many tear supplements are available, e.g. *g.* hypromellose 0.3%. *Oc.* simple and *oc.* Lacri-Lube provide longer lasting lubrication in cases of corneal exposure.

EYE EMERGENCIES

After a brief history and examination you should be able to categorize the emergency as shown in Table 8.1. The relevant history and examination for each category are given.

Blunt trauma

Lifesaving measures must take precedence but, when the integrity of an eye is in doubt, protect it with a hard shield (cartella) until a full ocular examination is possible.

History

Note the exact time and nature of the injury. Trauma inflicted during sports or assaults may cause both ocular and orbital injury. Shuttlecocks and squash balls 'fit' into the orbit and cause particularly severe ocular injuries. Record the nature of the pain: foreign body sensation occurs with corneal abrasions and conjunctival lacerations; aching often accompanies a hyphaema or microscopic hyphaema (in this case, a slit-lamp is required to detect the red blood cells suspended in the aqueous humour); paraesthesia over the gums

Table 8.1 Categorization of eye emergencies

- Trauma
  - Blunt
  - Penetrating or particulate
  - Chemical
  - Radiation
- Red eye (no history of trauma)
- Visual disturbance
  - Flashes and floaters
  - Visual loss
- Diplopia
- Lid disorders
  - Lid swelling
  - Lid malposition
  - Skin lesions

and cheek follows infraorbital nerve injury and is often associated with an orbital floor fracture. Blurred vision may result from a hyphaema or corneal injury. Flashes and floaters may occur following retinal injury.

Enquire about any previous ophthalmic history. Ocular surgery weakens the eye and increases the risk of globe rupture following blunt trauma. A long-standing history of retinal pathology or severe myopia (short sight) is associated with a higher risk of retinal detachment.

Examination

Note the presence of a periorbital haematoma. Examine lid lacerations carefully for involvement of the lid margin or lacrimal punctae which require urgent repair by an ophthalmologist. Ptosis may result from periorbital haematoma, rupture of the levator aponeurosis or oculomotor (third) nerve palsy secondary to intracranial injury. Palpate the skin overlying the orbit for surgical emphysema and test for hypoaesthesia over the cheek. If these signs are present, suspect an orbital floor (blow-out) fracture.

Bruising and swelling are rarely severe enough to prevent ocular examination – carefully part the lids using gauze, avoiding pressure on the globe (Fig. 8.4).

Assess the patient's eye movements. The combination of enophthalmos and impaired eye elevation strongly suggests a blow-out fracture. Visual acuity measurement should never be omitted. A large, poorly reacting pupil may result from either blunt trauma to the eye (traumatic mydriasis) or a third nerve palsy secondary to head trauma. An RAPD and red desaturation may result from traumatic optic neuropathy or from an extensive retinal detachment.

Document the anterior segment findings diagrammatically, noting the size and position of conjunctival and corneal abrasions and the height of a hyphaema in millimetres. Subconjunctival haemorrhages are common after trauma but the absence of a posterior limit to the haemorrhage should make you suspect a basal skull fracture. Black uveal pigment visible beneath the conjunctiva implies that the globe has been perforated or ruptured.

Do not use mydriatic agents for fundoscopy in cases of severe ocular trauma associated with visual disturbance until the case has been discussed with an ophthalmologist. An obscured red reflex may result from a hyphaema, cataract, vitreous haemorrhage or retinal detachment. Look for retinal haemorrhages and commotio retinae (an opalescent appearance secondary to traumatic retinal oedema). A retinal detachment appears as an convex, grey veil laced with blood vessels that obstructs the view beyond.

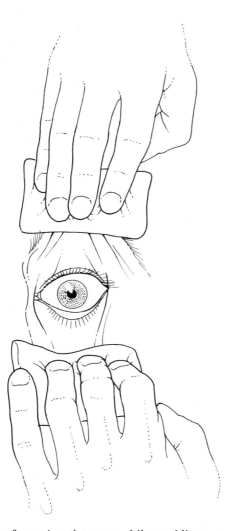

Fig. 8.4   Method of opening the eyes while avoiding pressure on the globe.

Management in the Accident and Emergency department

If you suspect the globe to be ruptured, protect the eye immediately with a hard shield. Keep the patient nil by mouth and try to prevent him/her from coughing or vomiting. Contact an ophthalmologist immediately. If urgent computed tomography is indicated for an associated cranial injury, request orbital sections in addition to intracranial imaging. This may spare the patient a return visit to the scanner.

Simple eye injuries secondary to blunt trauma may be treated by a non-specialist but if the diagnosis is in doubt or more serious pathology is present, urgent referral should be made. Corneal abrasions may be treated by the instillation of *g.* homatropine 2%, *oc.* chloramphenicol and overnight padding. Thereafter, a 4-day course of *g./oc.* chloramphenicol used four times daily provides adequate antibacterial prophylaxis. If the abrasion involves the central cornea or the patient is a contact lens wearer, review the eye every 24 hours until the epithelial defect has healed. Advise patients with peripheral abrasions to return should the symptoms worsen or last more than 48 hours. Consider tetanus prophylaxis in patients with skin lacerations; if peripheral to the orbital rim these may be sutured in the Accident and Emergency Department.

Penetrating or particulate trauma

High-velocity particles (generated when using hand or power tools) may penetrate the eye but often cause surprisingly little pain. Low-velocity impact with sharp objects (even the spine of a leaf) may cause corneal perforation.

History

Document the exact time of the injury, the material involved (e.g. iron, copper, glass or plant matter), its velocity and whether goggles were worn. The nature of associated pain assists in diagnosis: foreign-body sensation often occurs with a subtarsal or corneal foreign body; aching suggests a more serious injury.

Examination

Examine the lids for lacerations as previously outlined. Reduced visual acuity may result from a corneal abrasion on the visual axis or a penetrating eye injury. Remember that perfect visual acuity does not exclude a serious injury. Examine the symmetry of the pupil carefully: a distorted pupil suggests a penetrating injury. An RAPD may be present in a severe penetrating injury.

Exclude corneal perforation by examining the cornea, pupil and depth of the anterior chamber. Examine the conjunctiva carefully, particularly where subconjunctival haemorrhage is present, since this may obscure an underlying scleral laceration. Document the size and position of corneal abrasions or foreign bodies. Multiple linear, vertical abrasions affecting the superior third of the cornea suggest the presence of a subtarsal foreign body, so, provided the eye appears intact, evert the upper lid and look for the foreign body (Fig. 8.2).

Patients who have been struck in the eye by a high-velocity particle while not wearing eye protection should have careful fundoscopy and orbital X-rays. Unless definite signs of globe penetration are present, mydriatics should be instilled to facilitate fundoscopy in the Accident and Emergency Department. Penetrating trauma may induce vitreous inflammation or haemorrhage, which will obscure the red reflex. Look for an intraocular foreign body in the vitreous or on the retina.

Management in the Accident and Emergency Department

Suspected penetrating eye trauma should be managed in the same manner as already described for a ruptured globe.

Following instillation of a topical anaesthetic, small superficial foreign bodies may be removed from the conjunctiva or cornea with a moistened sterile cotton bud. Metallic foreign bodies often leave rust stains on the cornea; this residue may be carefully scraped off under slit-lamp magnification with a 25 gauge needle (or a burr). If a slit-lamp is unavailable, refer the patient to an ophthalmologist. Following removal of a subtarsal or small, non-central corneal foreign body prescribe *g./oc.* chloramphenicol four times daily for 4 days, prescribe oral analgesia if necessary and review if symptoms persist for longer than 48 hours. If the corneal foreign body is incompletely removed or central, apply *g.* homatropine and *oc.* chloramphenicol, pad the eye and review the patient every 24 hours to evaluate epithelial healing.

Chemical injury

Immediate irrigation for alkali (e.g. cements, plasters) and acid injuries can be sight-saving. Exposure to detergents and irritants (e.g. mace) also requires early copious irrigation. Fortunately, most cases receive some irrigation on site by first-aiders before transfer to hospital.

History

Take a brief history and record the nature of the chemical, the time of the accident and any first aid given. Chemical injuries are frequently bilateral. Start irrigating the eyes immediately; ocular examination should wait until this has been carried out.

Irrigation for chemical injuries

Lie the patient down with the head tilted towards the side to be irrigated; instil several drops of topical anaesthetic. Protect clothing with towels and position a kidney dish to receive the fluid, then direct a stream of isotonic saline from a 500 ml bag into the eye using a giving set. Irrigate the conjunctival fornices by everting the lids and remove any particles with a moistened cotton bud. Continue irrigation for 20 min. Allow 5 min for equilibration before checking the pH in the inferior fornix with litmus paper. If the pH is abnormal, continue irrigation until the pH is 7.

Examination

Examine the lids for burns, looking for involvement of the punctae. Use fluorescein to aid identification of conjunctival and corneal burns. Burns are often situated on the inferior half of the globe because Bell's reflex will have caused an upward rotation of the eye on lid closure. Corneal chemical burns range in severity from small spots of staining (punctate erosions) to large epithelial defects. Beware the very white eye following severe chemical injury since this indicates that extensive vascular occlusion has occurred. Conjunctival and corneal ischaemia are associated with a poor prognosis.

Management in the Accident and Emergency Department

All patients should undergo irrigation in the casualty department as previously described. Urgently refer all patients who have been exposed to alkaline or acidic chemicals to an ophthalmologist. If a patient has been exposed only to a mild irritant (e.g. detergent), and if the pH following irrigation is 7, the visual acuity is normal and only punctate erosions can be seen on the cornea, the patient may be treated in casualty. Instil *g.* homatropine 2% and *oc.* chloramphenicol and pad the worse eye. Prescribe oral analgesia and *g./oc.* chloramphenicol four times a day for 4 days, advising the patient to return for review if symptoms should last longer than 24 hours.

Radiation injury

The most common ocular radiation injury is 'arc eye'. Usually there is a specific history of welding or sunbed use without protective eyewear over the preceding 24 hours. Ultraviolet keratopathy results in severe bilateral foreign body sensation and photophobia. Examination findings include circumcorneal injection and multiple punctate erosions over the interpalpebral third of each cornea. Apply *g.* homatropine and *oc.* chloramphenicol, pad the worse of the two eyes, prescribe oral analgesia and ask the patient to return after 48 hours, if still symptomatic.

Thermal ocular injuries are less common, usually superficial and limited to the eyelids. Mild burns to the eyelids which do not involve the lacrimal punctae may be treated with *oc.* chloramphenicol for antibacterial prophylaxis. Patients with deep, severe facial burns may develop chemosis, resulting in corneal exposure, and should be referred to an ophthalmologist after admission.

RED EYE

This is probably the most frequent eye complaint encountered in either the Accident and Emergency Department or on the ward. Careful questioning about the onset of the symptoms and the associated features will give you a strong indication of the likely diagnosis. A thorough eye examination should confirm your suspicions.

History

Pain Severe **foreign body sensation** may result from corneal ulceration, erosions or loose surgical sutures. The pain and photophobia caused by a corneal ulcer typically increase in severity over several days. The ulcer may be sterile or microbial in nature; suspect a bacterial aetiology in wearers of soft contact lenses, the elderly and the infirm.

An uncomfortable, **gritty sensation** is commonly caused by blepharitis, dry eyes or conjunctivitis. A pterygium is an abnormal wing of conjunctiva that extends on to the nasal or temporal cornea. If raised on the ocular surface, the epithelial surface of the pterygium can dry and cause discomfort.

A mild, **bruised, tender sensation** is characteristic of episcleritis, while a more severe **ache** may occur with scleritis, uveitis or acute glaucoma. Anterior uveitis (iritis) causes an increasingly severe ache and photophobia and may occur recurrently in young adults. Acute glaucoma may result from primary closure of the drainage angle or as a complication of surgery or retinal vascular occlusion. Endophthalmitis is a devastating but uncommon intraocular infection which may occur after penetrating trauma, surgery or, more rarely, by haematogenous spread of infection.

A **painless, bright red eye** in which vascular markings are masked by blood is characteristic of subconjunctival haemorrhage. This condition may follow a Valsalva manoeuvre or occur spontaneously especially in hypertensive patients.

Discharge **Watery discharge** is an early feature of viral conjunctivitis, which is often associated with a cold or sore throat. Although the onset of viral conjunctivitis may be unilateral, the second eye inevitably becomes infected within days. **Mucoid discharge** may be associated with allergic conjunctivitis, which may be acute or seasonal.

Mucopurulent discharge is a feature of bacterial or chlamydial conjunctivitis.

Previous ophthalmic and medical history Patients who have ankylosing spondylitis, sarcoidosis or other connective tissue diseases are at risk of developing uveitis. A history of previous attacks of uveitis should increase your suspicion of another episode. Patients who develop a red, painful eye soon after eye surgery may have postoperative uveitis or endophthalmitis. Suture problems may occur in patients up to 2 years following cataract extraction.

Examination

The preauricular lymph nodes will be enlarged and tender in patients with viral or chlamydial conjunctivitis. Examine the lids: conjunctivitis causes the lids to be swollen but not erythematous; scaly lid margins with misdirected lashes are a sign of blepharitis. Evert the lids and examine the conjunctival fornices. The pattern of conjunctival vascular engorgement will aid the diagnosis: conjunctival injection in the fornices suggests conjunctivitis; circumcorneal injection may result from corneal ulceration, iritis or acute glaucoma; sectorial injection suggests peripheral corneal ulceration or episcleritis. Chemosis is suggestive of allergic conjunctivitis.

Always check the visual acuity. A painful, red eye with associated reduction in vision always requires referral to an ophthalmologist. Compare the size and shape of the pupils: iris spasm secondary to anterior uveitis makes the pupil in the affected eye smaller than its partner; the pupil may also be irregular because of the formation of adhesions between the iris and anterior lens surface (posterior synechiae); acute primary angle closure glaucoma classically results in a vertically oval pupil which is slightly larger than its partner.

Examine the cornea as previously described. A lustreless, misty cornea may result from acute glaucoma. Bacterial ulceration usually appears as a white, round lesion several millimetres in diameter. Herpetic ulceration typically produces a dendritic pattern on fluorescein staining. Punctate erosions result from dry eyes, blepharitis, viral conjunctivitis or recurrent erosion syndrome. A corneal abrasion in the absence of a history of trauma should make you look carefully for ingrowing eyelashes. Black corneal sutures, visible under the magnification of an ophthalmoscope, will stain with fluorescein if loose or broken. A hypopyon (a pus level in the anterior chamber) may be seen in bacterial keratitis or endophthalmitis and is a very serious finding.

Do not use mydriatics in the examination of patients with red, painful eyes unless the case has been discussed with an ophthalmologist.

Management in the Accident and Emergency Department

Some common conditions may be safely managed by non-specialists and the treatment is outlined below. However, if you are unsure of the diagnosis or suspect a more serious pathology you should arrange urgent referral. Infants, contact lens wearers and patients who have reduced visual acuity should be seen by an ophthalmologist. Contact lens wearers should be told to bring their solutions, lens case and lenses to the consultation. Patients who have had previous attacks of uveitis often recognize subsequent attacks and should be referred for slit-lamp examination even in the absence of signs on torch examination.

Advise patients with blepharitis to clean their lids at night-time with cotton buds dipped in a dilute baby shampoo solution and prescribe tear supplements and *oc.* simple to be applied to the lid margins at night. A patient presenting with a spontaneous subconjunctival haemorrhage should have his/her blood pressure checked. The dramatic appearance of the haemorrhage often worries the patient and reassurance should be given that the redness will resolve within a month. A severe bleed may cause the conjunctiva to prolapse and become dry, but regular *g.* hypromellose should relieve any discomfort.

Conjunctival swabs are not required for most cases of mild microbial conjunctivitis. Patients should be warned that the symptoms may initially worsen but should eventually resolve after several weeks. Prescribe *g.* chloramphenicol to be used four times daily over this period; cool compresses may provide symptomatic relief. Conjunctivitis is extremely contagious and patients should take precautions to prevent spread within the family. Cases of neonatal conjunctivitis require urgent referral to an ophthalmologist; cases of atypical or chronic conjunctivitis need less urgent review. Acute allergic conjunctivitis may be treated with saline irrigation of the conjunctival fornices in order to remove the offending allergen; cold compresses will reduce the associated lid swelling. Prescribe *g.* sodium cromoglycate or *g.* lodoxamide for patients with seasonal allergic conjunctivitis, to be used throughout the hay-fever season.

VISUAL DISTURBANCE

Most patients with visual disturbance will require referral to an ophthalmologist, the urgency being determined by your findings.

Flashes and floaters

History

Zigzag flashes and transient visual field defects may represent a migrainous aura. Unilateral flashes result from vitreous traction on the retina, often a result of involutional changes of the vitreous gel, causing it to detach from the retina. Floaters result from the movement of red blood cells (vitreous haemorrhage) or leucocytes (vitritis) within the vitreous cavity.

Visual loss

History

Transient visual loss Amaurosis fugax, a monocular, shutter-like visual field defect lasting from seconds to minutes, is caused by cholesterol emboli passing through the retinal circulation. A congested, swollen optic disc resulting from raised intracranial pressure (papilloedema) may cause transient visual loss on bending or coughing. Ischaemic optic neuropathy secondary to giant cell arteritis or atherosclerosis may initially cause transient loss of vision, but a permanent, often bilateral visual loss may occur within days or weeks as the blood supply of the optic nerve head eventually becomes occluded.

Subacute loss of vision Diabetic patients may complain of a shower of floaters, resulting in reduced vision. The common cause is a spontaneous vitreous haemorrhage secondary to proliferative diabetic retinopathy. Retinal vein occlusion is a common cause of field defect and blurred vision in middle-aged patients. Optic neuritis causes central visual loss in young adults and is often associated with pain on eye movement. Suspect a retinal detachment in patients with an initial history of flashes and floaters who have developed visual field loss and reduction in vision. Although patients with age-related macular degeneration usually suffer a gradual reduction in their reading vision, central vision can be lost quite abruptly following a macular haemorrhage.

Acute loss of vision Severe sudden loss of vision usually has an arterial cause. Occlusion of the retinal artery (central retinal artery occlusion) or the posterior ciliary arteries (anterior ischaemic optic neuropathy) may occur secondary to atherosclerosis or giant cell arteritis.

Gradual loss of vision Cataract and age-related macular degeneration characteristically cause gradual reduction in visual acuity. Cata-

Table 8.2 Reduction in vision: summary of examination findings

Condition	RAPD	Visual field	Optic nerve head	Retinal haemorrhages	Other features
Optic neuritis	Present	Central scotoma	Swollen/ normal	Peripapillary haemorrhages may be present	Variable reduction in visual acuity and pain on eye movement
Malignant hypertension	Absent	Enlarged blind spot	Swollen	Peripapillary	Bilateral with cotton wool spots, arteriovenous nipping and macular exudates
Papilloedema	Absent	Enlarged blind spot	Swollen	Peripapillary	Bilateral with cotton wool spots, engorged veins and disc hyperaemia
Anterior ischaemic optic neuropathy	Present	Altitudinal field loss	Swollen	Peripapillary	Suspect giant cell arteritis
Optic atrophy	Present	Central scotoma	Pale	Absent	Common end-point of optic nerve pathology
Branch retinal vein occlusion	Absent	Altitudinal or sectorial	Normal	Sectorial	Cotton wool spots present in sector of occlusion
Central retinal vein occlusion	Present (if severe)	Global reduction	Swollen	Extensive throughout posterior retina	Cotton wool spots; engorged, tortuous retinal veins
Central retinal artery occlusion	Present	Global reduction	Pale	Absent	Pale retina with cherry-red spot at the fovea, attenuated arterioles
Retinal detachment	Present (if extensive)	Initially peripheral	Normal	May occur near the tear	Flashers and floaters followed by a field defect; greyish veil of detached retina may be seen
Age-related macular degeneration	Absent	Central scotoma	Normal	Occasionally at the macular	Yellowish drusen and pigment clumping at the macula in elderly patients

racts typically cause the vision to be misty throughout the visual field whereas macular degeneration affects the central vision.

Previous ophthalmic and medical history   Patients with severe myopia or pre-existing retinal pathology have an increased risk of retinal detachment. Document conditions such as diabetes, hypertension and other cardiovascular risk factors. Question elderly patients with transient or acute loss of vision carefully for symptoms of giant cell arteritis such as headache, anorexia, temporal tenderness, jaw claudication and myalgia.

Examination

Examine the visual acuity and test the visual fields, RAPD and red desaturation.

All cases of recent visual disturbance require urgent ophthalmic referral and pupillary dilatation. You should dilate only the pupil of the affected eye so that the ophthalmologist can recheck the pupillary responses. Cataract and vitreous haemorrhage will obscure the red reflex while a retinal detachment will make it look grey. Assess the appearance of the disc and compare it to the other side. Retinal pallor and a cherry red spot at the fovea are the characteristic signs of ischaemia secondary to a central retinal artery occlusion. An early retinal detachment may be too peripheral to see with an ophthalmoscope but extension with time and gravity cause the detachment to become visible as a grey veil laced with blood vessels occluding the view of the fundus. The examination findings are summarized in Table 8.2.

Management in the Accident and Emergency Department

All patients with visual disturbance should have their blood pressure measured; test their urine for diabetes. Measure the ESR in patients over 50 years old who have symptoms suggestive of giant cell arteritis. Patients with classical migraine should be reassured and discharged to the care of their GP. Patients with bilateral disc swelling secondary to malignant hypertension or possibly raised intracranial pressure should be referred to a general physician and neurologist respectively for admission. Patients with unilateral disc swelling or recent disturbance of vision require urgent referral to an ophthalmologist. Discuss cases of chronic visual loss with an ophthalmologist so that an appropriate appointment for consultation can be made.

DIPLOPIA

History

Diplopia may be truly binocular or monocular. Monocular diplopia usually results from the scattering of light by a cataract and will continue to be present when the other eye is closed, whereas binocular diplopia will resolve when one eye is shut. An acute onset of binocular diplopia results often results from cranial nerve palsy, but other conditions such as myasthenia gravis, thyroid eye disease or decompensation of a childhood squint may cause similar symptoms. Ask the patient if the images are separated vertically or horizontally and if an object appears tilted when viewed by the eyes independently. Ascertain whether the diplopia is ever associated with a ptosis, is intermittent or worsens with fatigue.

Previous ophthalmic and medical history   Adults sometimes lose the ability to control a long-term squint – these patients will have a history of a childhood squint, which may have required surgical correction. Document a positive history of diabetes, hypertension or a thyroid disorder. Giant cell arteritis may cause cranial nerve palsies and patients should be carefully questioned for symptoms of the disease.

Examination

Examine the lids for a ptosis and measure the visual acuity. Compare the size and reactivity of the pupils and chart the eye movements as previously described. An oculomotor (third) nerve palsy results in a unilateral ptosis and in the visual axis being displaced downwards and laterally with reduced movement in every direction except abduction. Where the third nerve palsy is secondary to intracranial compression, e.g. posterior communicating artery aneurysm, the pupil will be dilated and unreactive. A trochlear (fourth) nerve palsy results in rotation (extortion) and elevation of the visual axis. The defect in ocular motility can be difficult to identify but suspect a fourth nerve palsy if the patient has vertical diplopia and is finding reading especially difficult. An abducent (sixth) nerve palsy results in the visual axis being displaced medially with limitation of abduction. Graves disease or an orbital pathology such as a blow-out fracture may restrict the upward movement of the eye both in abduction and adduction.

Management in the Accident and Emergency Department

Patients with an acute onset of diplopia should have their blood pressure measured; test for diabetes. If there are symptoms of giant cell arteritis, take blood for measurement of the ESR. Patients who have a third nerve palsy involving the pupil should be urgently referred to a neurosurgeon; all other patients with diplopia should be seen by an ophthalmologist urgently.

EYELID DISORDERS

Although most lid problems are a harmless nuisance, more serious orbital and intracranial conditions may initially present with lid signs.

Lid swelling

Localized swelling

A **stye** is an infected eyelash follicle that causes an erythematous swelling at the lid margin. Most styes will resolve spontaneously within a fortnight but hot compresses and application of *oc.* chloramphenicol four times daily may speed the process.

The oil-secreting meibomian glands are enclosed within the tarsal plates. Blockage of the duct and subsequent infection of the inspissated oil results in an erythematous, tender swelling in the tarsal plate called a **meibomian cyst**. Treatment is similar to that described for a stye, but a hard lump (**chalazion**) often persists and requires incision and curettage by an ophthalmologist.

Generalized swelling

Preseptal cellulitis is an infection of the lids superficial to the orbital septum and may develop after trauma or from a previously localized lid infection (e.g. meibomian cyst). Although malaise and pyrexia may be associated symptoms, preseptal cellulitis never involves the globe or optic nerve. Patients with preseptal cellulitis should be referred urgently to an ophthalmologist but admission is not usually required. **Orbital cellulitis** is a potentially fatal infection of the orbit which presents with generalized, erythematous lid swelling and pyrexia. Orbital cellulitis usually occurs in children who have pre-existing sinusitis or dental infection. The presence of proptosis, restricted eye movements, reduced vision and RAPD are important features that distinguish orbital cellulitis from the less serious preseptal cellulitis. Refer patients with orbital cellulitis for admission for intravenous antibiotic therapy and CT scan, under the care of an ophthalmologist or paediatrician.

An acute onset of non-erythematous lid swelling associated with intense itching and chemosis is a common feature of acute allergic conjunctivitis following exposure to an allergen.

Lid malposition

Entropion (inversion of the lid margin) is common in the elderly. Corneal abrasions from the inturned lashes may be prevented by everting the lid with tape applied vertically from cheek to lid margin. After excluding corneal ulceration, prescribe *oc.* chloramphenicol to be used four times daily for lubrication and antibacterial prophylaxis and refer the patient for elective lid surgery. **Ectropion** (eversion of the lid margin) may be secondary to ageing or a facial (seventh) nerve palsy. The everted lid position causes epiphora and requires routine surgical correction.

Skin lesions

Herpes simplex virus commonly causes vesicular lid lesions associated with localized oedema. Perform a thorough ocular examination to exclude Herpes simplex keratitis. Acyclovir ointment may be used five times daily on the skin lesions. If there is any evidence of ocular involvement, refer the patient to an ophthalmologist.

Shingles frequently occurs in the territory of the ophthalmic division of the trigeminal (fifth) nerve and is called herpes zoster ophthalmicus. It causes a strictly unilateral, vesicular rash over the forehead, upper eyelid and nose and may cause serious ocular complications such as keratitis and uveitis. Most ophthalmologists would recommend the use of oral acyclovir 800 mg five times daily if initiated within 72 hours of the onset of the rash. A slit-lamp examination by an ophthalmologist is required should the eye become red, sore or photophobic.

OCULAR PROBLEMS ON NEUROSURGICAL AND ENT WARDS

Proptosis

Proptosis results from a rise in intraorbital pressure, which may occur secondary to space-occupying lesions in the orbit (e.g. maxillary, nasopharyngeal and primary orbital tumours) or from immunologically mediated swelling of the orbital contents (e.g. thyroid eye disease). Complications include corneal exposure keratitis and optic nerve compression. Early detection of these complications by regular examination may prevent blindness. This should include: regular testing of visual acuity, pupillary reactions (for an RAPD), testing for red desaturation and fluorescein examination of the cornea. If the proptosis is mild, prescribe *g.* hypromellose regularly throughout the day and *oc.* simple at night; if severe, apply *oc.* simple and tape the eye day and night by positioning a 5 cm strip of porous tape horizontally over the manually approximated lid margins. Patients should be urgently reviewed by an ophthalmologist if there are signs of optic nerve compression or exposure keratitis. High-dose steroids, orbital radiotherapy or decompression may be indicated for optic nerve compression and tarsorrhaphy or ptosis induction for corneal exposure.

Facial (seventh) nerve palsy

A lower motor neurone facial nerve palsy may follow neurosurgical procedures (e.g. acoustic neuroma excision) or compression from inner ear or intracranial tumours, or it may be idiopathic (Bell's palsy). Paralysis of orbicularis oculi results in lagophthalmos (inability to close the eyelids) and corneal exposure, especially if the cornea is insensitive or Bell's reflex (p. 158) is absent. These signs should be documented at the initial examination. Subsequently, perform regular examination of the cornea with fluorescein. If corneal sensation is normal and the palsy is thought to be temporary, prescribe *g.* hypromellose to be applied every 2 hours during the day and *oc.* simple to be used before the lids are taped at night. If corneal sensation is absent, the cornea is ulcerated or the palsy is likely to be permanent, urgently refer the patient to an ophthalmologist – a tarsorrhaphy or ptosis induction (with botulinum toxin) may be indicated.

Postoperative painful red eye

Inadvertent exposure of an eye during surgery under general anaesthesia may result in a painful corneal erosion. An epithelial defect that takes up fluorescein stain will be present on ocular examination. Instil *g.* homatropine, *oc.* chloramphenicol and pad the eye. If the corneal epithelium is not healed within 24 hours the patient should be referred to an ophthalmologist.

Plastic surgery

9

Andrew D. Wilmshurst

Plastic surgery is predominantly concerned with repair and reconstruction of the skin and soft tissues: the restoration of form and function. This chapter will concentrate on techniques applicable to the correction of injury, disease or deformity of the skin, where these are likely to cross the path of the surgeon in training.

SKIN CLOSURE

When you suture a wound aim to produce a tidy linear closure with minimal tension on the skin sutures while avoiding the complications of haematoma, infection and dehiscence.

It is important not to close the wound by placing undue tension on the skin sutures. Reduce tension where necessary by using buried absorbable sutures through the deep layer of the dermis. Use 3/0 or 4/0 Vicryl or Dexon and invert the suture so that the knot lies on the deep aspect. It should be emphasized that these are dermal sutures supporting skin closure, not fat sutures, which are of doubtful value in any type of wound closure. Many smaller wounds, particularly on the face, close easily without the need for buried sutures.

Undermining the wound margins to aid closure is an overrated technique. The extra dissection and increased dead-space aggravate the risk of haematoma, and the gain in mobility of the wound edges is negligible except in areas of firmly tethered skin such as the nose or fingertip.

After an extensive excision which leaves significant dead space on closure, leave a small suction drain and remove it after a few hours.

Suturing of the skin itself to complete a tidy wound closure requires accuracy and gentleness. These standards are easier to attain if the instruments you use are fine and in good condition.

Provided that tension across the wound has been largely neutralized, the skin sutures are required simply to appose the two margins as near perfectly as possible, thus allowing optimum primary healing to take place. Use fine sutures to impart sensitivity in handling and tying, and space them closely and evenly to obtain accurate apposition. Monofilament synthetic non-absorbable material produces no tissue reaction and makes better quality scars than braided natural materials. Within this range the softness and flexibility of polybutester give excellent knotting characteristics and in addition this suture is swaged on to very sharp reverse-cutting needles ideal for delicate skin surgery. Equally acceptable to many surgeons are polypropylene or nylon. Use 5/0 or 6/0 gauge for the face, placing sutures approximately 3 mm from the margin and 3 mm apart.

Avoid inversion of the wound margins, which results in delayed wound healing or an ugly scar, or both. Aim for slight eversion, obtaining a 'square' bite of tissue with the curved needle (Fig. 9.1).

Put the needle into the skin at a right angle, take a broad section of dermis and subcutaneous tissue, enter the opposite margin at an equal depth in the wound and bring it out from the skin on the other side at the same angle and an equal distance from the margin. Correct passage of the needle can be aided by everting the skin edge with a fine hook or a pair of forceps. Tie the suture gently to com-

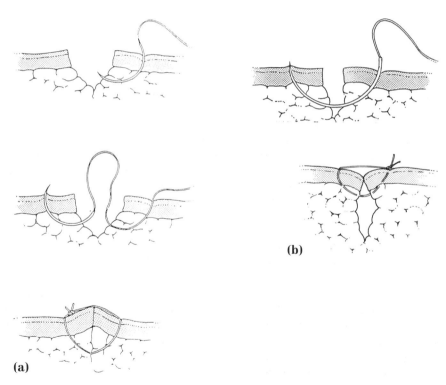

(b)

(a)

Fig. 9.1 Techniques of simple suture. **(a)** 'Square' bite produces moderate eversion and sound closure. **(b)** Shallow oblique bite produces inversion and faulty healing.

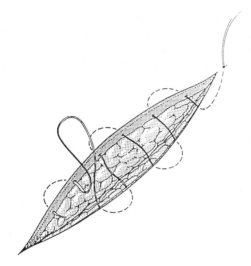

Fig. 9.2   Continuous subcuticular suture.

press the deep tissues and produce a degree of pouting of the skin edge.

Tie the knots using the needle holder. Synthetic monofilament sutures require four throws for security. Obtaining a perfect wound closure is a matter of practice and experience. Techniques that will help you in this include differential tension on the two ends of the suture while snugging down the knot, or gentle pressure on one side of the wound with the tip of the needle holder while tying.

Avoid at all costs excessive tension in the suture with strangulation of tissue. Take into account postoperative swelling which will develop during the first 48 hours, but weigh this against fluid already in the tissues from infiltrated local anaesthetic. Generally speaking tighten the suture just enough to bring the wound margins into contact but no more.

In the thin loose skin on the dorsum of hand or foot, mattress sutures may be required to ensure eversion. At other sites on the limbs and trunk, use a continuous subcuticular suture. These can be left in place for 3 weeks, or permanently if absorbable, and eliminate the risk of leaving suture marks. Use 3/0 or 4/0 polypropylene, taking advantage of its high tensile strength and low drag properties, which are required in a pull-out suture. Take small bites with the curved cutting needle, running horizontally from side to side at a constant mid-dermal depth (Fig. 9.2).

Insert the needle opposite to or just back from the point at which it has emerged from the opposite wound edge. In a long wound, bring the suture out as a loop across the wound every 10 cm to enable it to be easily removed in sections (see Chapter 1). Avoid subcuticular sutures on the face as it is more difficult to achieve exact apposition with this technique.

The timing of suture removal

This is determined by the balance of two conflicting interests: the necessity to support the wound until skin healing is secure against the concern to avoid permanent suture marks. The factors that may contribute to the ugly crosshatched appearance often seen in scars include excessive tension in the stitches, infection of the wound and the region of the body in which the wound lies. However, the single most important influence is the length of time for which the suture is left in place: 7 days appears to be the safe limit for avoidance of these marks. Stitches on the face may be removed in most cases by the fifth day, and earlier than this in young children. On the trunk and limbs a minimum of 10–14 days is usually required, and there is thus an advantage in using a subcuticular suture.

EXCISION OF SKIN LESIONS

Operating sessions for excision of minor skin lesions or 'lumps and bumps' are often located in an outpatient department, where conditions may fall short of the ideal. There are, however, certain requirements which represent the minimum that is acceptable.

The patient should be positioned on a table or trolley adjustable for height and tilt. A hand table must be available for operations on the upper limb, and stools for the surgeon and assistant. It is important that both surgeon and patient are comfortable and relaxed. The whole session will move faster and more efficiently if there is a nurse to scrub and assist as well as a circulating nurse. A proper operating theatre light is essential.

Instrument sets for minor surgery should be designed to suit the type of delicate excisional procedures involved, and should not be collections of oddments and cast-offs. A large number of instruments is not required, but they should be fine, sharp and have tips that meet. A typical list will include:

- Small needle holder (5 inch)
- Scalpel handle, to take a No. 15 blade
- Two pairs of toothed Adson's forceps, one coarse, one fine

- Two skin hooks
- Two catspaw retractors
- Small curved dissecting scissors
- Iris scissors
- Small suture scissors
- Two fine curved mosquito forceps
- Bipolar diathermy.

Planning the incision

Excise small lesions in the skin or on its surface with a segment of immediately adjacent skin, to obtain a tidy direct closure. Make a 'surgical ellipse', actually a lenticular shape with pointed ends, three to four times as long as it is wide, to avoid heaping up of the skin at each end when it is closed.

Correct orientation of the ellipse is important so that the resulting scar lies in the line of local skin creases. On the face these lines correspond to the age wrinkles or the creases caused by facial expression (Fig. 9.3).

On the rest of the body identify the 'relaxed skin tension lines' by gently pinching the skin in different directions until you identify the

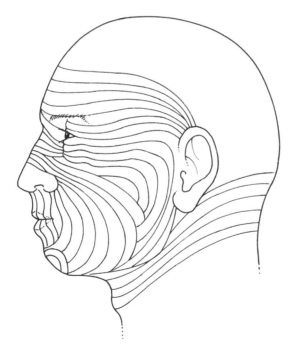

Fig. 9.3 Lines of relaxed skin tension on the face.

pinch done with the least resistance which produces the longest and clearest skin creases. Align the ellipse parallel to these creases. Langer's lines are not relevant, and do not attempt to memorize lines of election, except perhaps on the face.

Excise skin lesions, particularly malignant ones, lying close to the free margin of features such as the lip, pinna, or eyelid, as a full thickness wedge of tissue so that closure, in two or three layers, produces a linear scar at right angles to the margin with minimal distortion.

Using a disposable mapping pen, draw the outline of the excision before injecting the local anaesthetic to avoid distortion. Allow several millimetres of normal skin as a safe margin around any lesion suspicious of malignancy. If you mark the lines of incision in this manner before cutting you can then proceed in a relaxed and confident manner.

Technique of excision

Infiltrate 0.5% lignocaine with adrenaline 1:200 000 solution, except in the digits or penis, where you must use lignocaine without adrenaline. A sensory nerve block may sometimes be appropriate in the face, but local infiltration has the advantages of a quicker onset of action, is more reliable in inexperienced hands and gives a drier field as a result of vasoconstriction due to the adrenaline. Reduce the pain of the injection by warming the solution beforehand, and infiltrate slowly. Ensure that the field has been adequately anaesthetized; a patient who suddenly feels pain half way through the procedure will lose confidence drastically.

Using a size 15 blade, incise the previously marked ellipse, making sure that the cuts are absolutely vertical. Include a generous portion of underlying fat from each pole of the ellipse to help to avoid the raised mounds or 'dog-ears' that may appear on closure. Unless clear alternative policies exist, send all specimens for histological examination.

Haemostasis will have been achieved to a substantial extent by the adrenaline in the local anaesthetic. Place a swab over the wound and wait for a further 60 seconds and then use the bipolar diathermy to coagulate remaining bleeding points, but do not be too obsessive. A minor capillary ooze is acceptable as closure progresses. Artery forceps are almost never required.

EXCISION OF SUBCUTANEOUS LESIONS

Small subcutaneous cysts and tumours are easily removed under a local anaesthetic in the same manner as cutaneous lesions. Infiltrate deep to the lesion as well as around it. Larger masses will leave behind significant dead space; do not hesitate to use a miniature suction drain left in place for a few hours. Remove it before the patient goes home.

Epidermal (sebaceous) cysts

Remove these with a narrow ellipse of overlying skin including the estimated site of the punctum, whether you can see it or not. Do not make a great effort to remove the cyst intact. Success is unlikely unless it is a pilar cyst on the scalp. When it ruptures express the contents and then remove the sac using blunt and sharp dissection. Complete removal may be particularly difficult if the cyst has previously been inflamed, infected or ruptured, but is nevertheless important, for any remnant left behind will predispose to wound infection and later recurrence. An infected cyst should not be operated upon unless simple incision and drainage are required. Treat it with an antibiotic and leave it until all trace of inflammation and induration has resolved.

Lipoma

A lipoma is removed through a simple skin crease incision. Frequently, especially on the limbs this can be kept quite short and the lipoma can be 'popped out' by squeezing it firmly between the finger tips. However, a lipoma that has been subject over many years to repeated trauma or pressure, for instance on the back, may require careful dissection to separate it from the surrounding fibrosis. Deeper subfascial or intermuscular lipomas usually require a general anaesthetic.

REPAIR OF FACIAL LACERATIONS

Assessment

Facial injuries caused by high-energy impacts require careful neurological and skeletal assessment, including the cervical spine. Exclude more severe injuries elsewhere. Neurosurgical, maxillofacial or ophthalmological opinions should be sought if necessary, before approaching repair of the skin and soft tissues. Unless they are the cause of airway obstruction or major haemorrhage, facial lacerations have low priority and may be left in some circumstances for up to 72 hours if, for example, other factors prevent safe general anaesthesia.

Anaesthesia

Simple lacerations may be dealt with using local anaesthetic with adrenaline. However, the instruments available in accident departments are often inappropriate for fine repair of facial wounds, and lighting and assistance may also be less than adequate unless a fully equipped minor operations theatre is available. The main operating theatre is usually the best place to repair these injuries.

Repair lacerations of any degree of complexity under a general anaesthetic, and then admit the patient overnight.

In children you may be able to close the wound using skin tapes or glue, provided that the wounds are minor, the site is suitable and there is no indication for exploration.

Exploration

Look specifically for:

- **areas of tissue loss**: animal or human bites, or areas of deep abrasion in road accidents, are common causes. Swelling and skin retraction frequently give rise to a false appearance of tissue loss. Systematically reappose the wound margins to correct the illusion.
- **traumatic elevation of skin flaps**: this is common in windscreen injuries and applies typically to the forehead and scalp. Elevate all flaps and explore the depths for foreign bodies and fractures before you replace the flap and repair the skin.
- **ingrained dirt**: remove the dirt with a scrubbing brush; excise it if it is resistant. If left it will produce permanent tattooing of the scar.
- **lacerations that cross feature lines or borders**: ensure that you obtain correct alignment of structures such as the vermilion border of the lip, the margin of the nostril or the line of the eyebrow, to avoid the severe cosmetic defect of a step deformity.
- **'through-and-through' penetrating wounds** into the mouth or nose or across the eyelid.
- **damage to the facial nerve or the parotid duct** in deep lacerations of the lateral portion of the cheek.

Debridement

Excise human bites and wounds that are heavily contaminated or more than 48 hours old. Open animal bites on the face need not be excised if they are fresh and minimally contused. Clean them thoroughly and treat the patient with systemic antibiotics. Excise skin flaps that are clearly non-viable, but conserve skin that is contused and possibly viable. The face has an extremely rich subdermal vascular plexus and these areas can be expected to survive. Remove all dirt.

Repair

Where possible convert oblique shelving lacerations caused by glass to vertical wounds by excision of their sloping margins, to prevent formation of broad, heaped-up scars. In a similar way and for the same reason the small C-shaped flaps produced by shattered windscreen glass can often be excised completely as ellipses and closed as straight wounds.

Division of the parotid duct or major branches of the facial nerve require expert repair using magnification and should be referred to an appropriate surgeon.

Repair large areas of tissue loss whose margins cannot be excised and closed primarily with a split skin graft. In the weeks following healing this will contract considerably, facilitating future reconstruction. Avulsion of a portion of the pinna may expose torn cartilage, which should be trimmed until the skin edges can be approximated. Reconstruction of these parts, at a later date, is technically demanding and not always feasible. Do not make promises to the patient along these lines at this time.

A laceration through the full thickness of the cheek or lip requires careful repair in layers, using 4/0 chromic catgut to mucosa and muscle, and an appropriate skin suture. Refer perforating eyelid injuries to an ophthalmic or plastic surgeon.

Repair facial lacerations using the suturing techniques described above. Buried dermal sutures are not usually required. Realign landmarks accurately, using interrupted 5/0 or 6/0 monofilament sutures. Have the sutures removed at 4–5 days.

METHODS OF OBTAINING SKIN COVER

Where a defect is too large to close directly, there is a progression of options available in the planning of how a healed wound is to be achieved. This is known as the 'reconstructive ladder' and commences on the bottom rung with the option of allowing the wound to heal spontaneously by epithelialization. From there one ascends mentally through a series of increasingly sophisticated techniques until the correct method for the particular patient and his wound is identified. Some of the simpler yet more versatile techniques are included here.

Split skin grafts

The advantages of split skin grafting are ease and versatility. Disadvantages include subsequent contraction of the graft, susceptibility to breakdown and a poor cosmetic appearance.

Anaesthesia

Small grafts may be taken under local anaesthetic, using an infiltration technique, a nerve block or local anaesthetic cream applied in copious quantities at least 2 hours before the procedure. If a large graft is required, and particularly if there is preliminary surgery to be done at the recipient site, use a general or regional anaesthetic.

Technique

Identify a suitable donor site, usually on the thigh, although other common sites are the upper outer arm or the buttock. The area should be shaved.

The Watson skin graft knife has a long, disposable blade mounted behind an adjustable bar which both protects the blade and determines the depth of cut and thickness of the graft. Adjustment, using the wheel at each end of the bar, is best done 'by eye' while holding the knife up to the light and observing the gap between blade and bar, although there is a scale on the instrument which may be used if preferred. For very small grafts use the Silver knife (Fig. 9.4), which carries a razor blade. Powered dermatomes are reserved for rapid harvesting of large areas of graft, as in the surgery of large burns.

Successful harvesting of a satisfactory sheet of skin depends on two principal factors. The first is an able assistant, whose task is to keep the area of skin under tension by employing one hand to grasp the thigh from beneath while the other hand holds a wooden board firmly edge down on the skin behind the advancing Watson knife. Lubricate the skin well with liquid paraffin. Maintain skin tension by advancing a board or the palm of your other hand across the skin in front of the blade.

The second factor is a relaxed and confident approach in taking the graft. Very little forward pressure is required. Allow the blade to do the work. Use a rapid to and fro action and hold the knife in a plane almost parallel with the skin (Fig. 9.5).

Dress the donor area with alginate sheets soaked in a dilute solution of bupivacaine in saline. Use plenty of gauze on top of this followed by a firm crepe bandage. This dressing should then be left intact for 10–14 days.

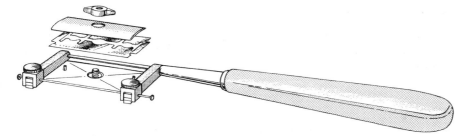

Fig. 9.4   The Silver knife.

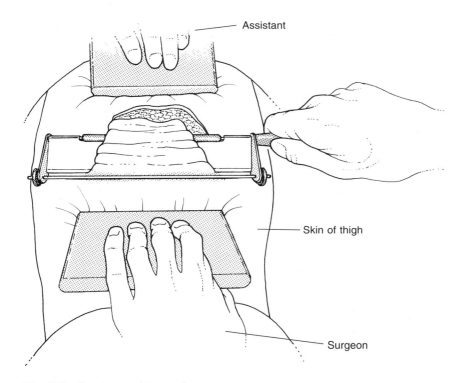

Fig. 9.5   Cutting a skin graft.

Applying the graft

Unless the graft is being applied to the face, it should be meshed before application. The introduction of machine-meshed grafts has been a minor revolution in skin grafting in recent years. The mesher converts the graft into a net with evenly spaced perforations. These allow the free egress of blood and serum, increase flexibility and conformity of the graft to irregular surfaces and permit overall expansion of the graft area. The mesh need only be expanded if a gain in area is required to fill the defect. The 'take' of these grafts is notably more reliable than that of unmeshed grafts.

Lay the graft on to the recipient bed and mould it into any irregularities. You may anchor the margins with sutures, staples or glue. Apply a bulky dressing such as plastic foam sponge over a layer of paraffin gauze under firm bandaging or adhesive strapping. This is not primarily a pressure dressing but is protective and to some degree splints the soft tissues to neutralize shearing forces.

In areas such as the trunk where there is difficulty in achieving a secure and stable graft dressing, the graft may be applied and exposed on the ward a day or two after the operation. It needs no securing if the patient is cooperative, and it can be observed and tended as necessary as it rapidly adheres to its bed and becomes stable. This technique requires a degree of nursing commitment. A dressing may be applied at night for protection during sleep. Grafts managed in this way have to be stored until used. Do this in theatre by wrapping the harvested skin in saline-moistened gauze, place it in a labelled sterile container and keep it in the ward refrigerator at 4°C.

If the graft has been dressed, carry out the first dressing change at 5–7 days. Trim and clean the graft before reapplying a protective dressing.

Pretibial flap laceration

Avulsion of a flap of skin and fat from the shin is a common injury resulting from relatively trivial accidents. Its clinical importance is mainly confined to the elderly where the skin is not only fragile but often very thin and with a poor blood supply. Steroid therapy exacerbates the problem.

Distally based flaps seldom survive when simply taped back into place. These injuries are frequently undertreated, resulting in an enormous waste of patient's and nurses' time as a prolonged period of repeated dressings finally concludes in the realization that a chronic ulcer has formed and that a skin graft is indicated. Where there is a significant area of damaged skin whose viability is in question, or where underlying fat has been disrupted or displaced by haematoma, formal debridement and immediate cover with a split skin graft is indicated. This need not be regarded as a major procedure, but may be carried out on an outpatient basis if suitable facilities exist.

Anaesthesia

In the elderly carry out the procedure under local anaesthesia, unless the injury is unusually extensive. Spinal anaesthesia may be appropriate in some cases.

Cover the skin graft donor site on the ipsilateral thigh with a generous quantity of local anaesthetic cream at least 2 hours before operation. Infiltrate the lacerated area with 10–20 ml of 0.5% lignocaine or bupivacaine with 1 : 200 000 adrenaline.

Technique

Excise all skin that has been elevated from its deep attachments. There are frequently fragments of loose fat within the zone of trauma. Debride these carefully until only firmly attached, healthy tissue remains. Often the injury through the fat extends to the deep fascia and in these cases it is better to excise the whole area of damaged fat and skin graft directly on to deep fascia. Secure haemostasis with bipolar diathermy. Take the skin graft with a Watson knife set for a very thin graft, to avoid the complication of a full-thickness defect arising at the donor site in this susceptible group of patients. Mesh the graft at a ratio of 1.5 : 1 and lay it in place with its margins overlapping the edges of the defect. Cyanoacrylate glue may be used to anchor the graft.

These patients are to be mobilized early, so ensure a secure dressing. Apply one layer of paraffin gauze followed by a piece of plastic foam sponge cut a little larger than the area of the graft. Then enclose the whole of the lower leg from toes to knee in a generous layer of orthopaedic wool bandage, apply a firm 10 cm crepe bandage and tape it securely.

Mobilize the patient as soon as s/he returns to the ward and send him/her home within 24 hours if s/he is safe on his/her feet and has some help at home. Arrange to see the patient again 6–7 days later and carry out the first graft dressing. Following this the limb will need firm elastic support for 3 months until the graft is mature and the leg is free of oedema.

In summary, the principles of the management of these injuries in the elderly are: immediate recognition and treatment on the day of injury, thorough debridement, a meshed skin graft firmly supported, and early mobilization and discharge.

The venous leg ulcer

A number of patients with venous ulcers are referred to the surgeon after a variety of conservative measures have failed to produce healing. A split skin graft simply laid on to the clean, granulating ulcer bed will often take satisfactorily, but long-term survival of the graft is more dependable if the ulcer is excised before grafting. There is no place for pinch grafting.

Preparation

Admit the patient a few days before the operation if there is marked oedema of the limb, inflammation of the surrounding skin or infected slough on the ulcer. Insist on bedrest, elevation of the leg and frequent dressing changes, and send swabs for bacteriology. Give narrow-spectrum antibiotics effective against Gram-positive cocci if cellulitis is present. Surgery may proceed once the leg is 'quiet' and the ulcer is relatively clean. Under these conditions colonization with organisms such as *Pseudomonas* or *Staphylococcus* may be ignored. On the other hand, the beta-haemolytic streptococcus, particularly Group A, will destroy a skin graft; avoid operating in the presence of this organism.

Technique

Under general or spinal anaesthesia, excise the whole ulcer tangentially using the Watson knife adjusted to a very 'thick' setting. Repeat this up to three or four slices until the ulcer and its bed are completely removed. It is important to clear the underlying layer of brown haemosiderin pigmentation. As this is removed a surface of clean white fibrous tissue is revealed. A graft will take readily on to this, but unless bone is about to be encountered it is advisable to go even deeper until either deep fascia or muscle is reached. Skin grafts on this tissue stand a reasonable chance of prolonged survival.

Subfascial ligation of perforating veins should be considered where there is clinical evidence of incompetent underlying perforators, a history of deep venous thrombosis or a particularly recalcitrant ulcer. The procedure may be done at the same time as the skin grafting and is appropriate for both medial and lateral ulcers. Make a longitudinal incision through the ulcer 2 cm behind the tibia medially or over the line of the fibula laterally. The incision is taken straight down through the deep fascia on to muscle belly. It should extend proximally as a fasciotomy right across the zone of circumferential constrictive fibrosis that is frequently present. Do not open any plane superficial to the deep fascia. Instead, elevate this fascia anteriorly and posteriorly and identify the perforating veins (with accompanying arteries) deep to it. Ligate the larger ones; small veins may be safely diathermied before dividing them.

Take split-skin grafts using the ipsilateral thigh as the donor site to confine the surgical field to one leg. Take a fresh Watson knife, cut medium-thickness grafts and mesh them. Glue, staple or suture the grafts in place and tuck a graft down into the furrow of the fasciotomy wound if one is present.

Apply a non-adherent and well-padded dressing wrapped in a firm crepe bandage. Confine the patient to bed for 4–5 days until the first graft dressing. If the take is good, allow mobilization to proceed, maintaining good elastic support to the whole limb below the knee.

To reduce the risk of these ulcers breaking down again in future years, advise the patient to continue with lifelong elastic support.

Full-thickness skin grafts

The versatility of full-thickness grafts is limited by their restricted size and reduced readiness to take on to a bed that is less than ideal. However, the lack of graft contraction and the relatively good cosmetic appearance make them acceptable for the repair of facial defects resulting from tumour excision, trauma or burns, and their durability is of value in hand surgery.

Donor sites

Since by definition the full depth of the skin is taken, direct closure of the donor site is required to allow primary healing. This is the only factor limiting the size of graft available; choose a site where the skin is relatively loose and closure can be obtained with an inconspicuous scar. Grafts to the face are taken from areas of similar skin quality, such as the postauricular sulcus, the preauricular area, the root of the neck on the posterior triangle, and the upper eyelid (for grafts to the opposite eyelid) (Fig. 9.6). Take larger grafts to other areas of the body from the inguinal crease, the antecubital fossa or the upper medial aspect of the arm.

Anaesthesia

The commonest application for these grafts is in the repair of defects on the face created by excision of small skin tumours. Local anaesthesia is appropriate for most of these operations. Use lignocaine with adrenaline and infiltrate both excision and donor sites after marking the margins of excision. Infiltrate even if general anaesthesia is being used, as this will reduce bleeding and will eliminate the need for systemic analgesia.

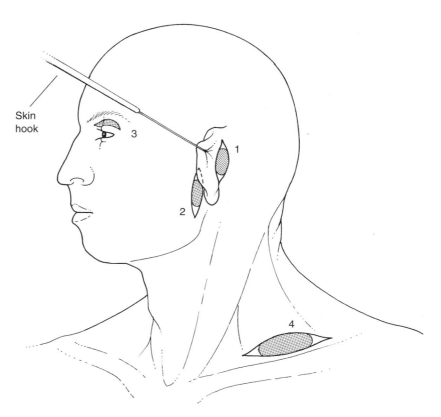

Skin hook

Fig. 9.6 Donor sites for full-thickness grafts to the face: 1. postauricular; 2. preauricular; 3. upper eyelid; 4. supraclavicular.

Technique

Excise the lesion and send it for histopathology. Obtain perfect haemostasis using the bipolar diathermy, for the graft will fail if lifted from its bed by haematoma.

Full-thickness grafts allow little margin for error in size and shape and should therefore be mapped out carefully. Either measure the defect with a ruler or make an exact pattern of it with a piece of sterile paper from the instrument trolley. Transfer this to the selected donor site and draw around it to map out the graft. Convert the shape into an ellipse in the skin crease line by adding a triangle at each end. Raise the graft using a No. 15 blade and a skin hook. With care, elevate the skin by sharp dissection leaving all the subcutaneous fat behind. Trim away and discard the triangle at each end and temporarily store the graft in a saline swab. Close the donor site with a few dermal 4/0 absorbable sutures and a subcuticular 4/0 polypropylene.

Turn your attention now to the excision site and check for complete haemostasis. Suture the graft into place with 4/0 silk sutures, leaving one end of each suture long. Cover the graft with a single layer of paraffin gauze cut to size and then apply a bulky bolus dressing of flavine wool or plastic foam sponge and tie the long ends of the silk over this to hold it firmly in place (Fig. 9.7).

This tie-over dressing initially provides some compression and helps to avoid haematoma but the pressure dissipates within a few hours and its main function thereafter is as a protective splint for the graft. Remove the dressing and sutures after 6–8 days.

Skin flaps

Definition

Flap cover represents a step above skin grafts on the reconstructive ladder. Unlike grafts, a flap is vascularized, the vessels passing through the base of the flap, or pedicle. This feature allows the transfer of a block of tissue rather than the thin sheet of skin that comprises a graft. Flaps are described or classified from a number of aspects, including the geometry of transfer, the distance of transfer, the anatomy of the arterial supply and the component tissues. They range in complexity from simple local skin flaps with a random blood supply to large blocks of tissue including muscle and bone transferred 'free' and revascularized microsurgically at the recipient site.

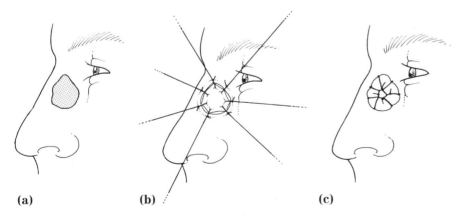

(a)   **(b)**   **(c)**

Fig. 9.7 Full-thickness skin grafts: tie-over technique. **(a)** the excised defect. **(b)** Graft sutured in place. **(c)** Tie-over completed.

Applications

- To cover important but relatively avascular structures such as bone, cartilage, joint and tendon. Not only do these tissues fail to accept a skin graft, but they also require good quality cover in terms of mobility and durability.
- Where quality of appearance is paramount: on the face.
- To prevent a contracture caused by scarring, or to correct one already present.
- To restore or maintain soft-tissue contour or provide cushioning over bony points.

Flap design

Having designed the flap, and before putting knife to skin, ask yourself some important final questions.

- What is the blood supply to the flap? Is it random or through a recognized vascular pedicle? Is it necessary to identify the vessels?
- Is the geometry correct? Will the flap reach where it is intended to?
- Is the flap large enough to fill the defect?
- Will the donor defect close directly, and in the line of the skin creases?
- What is the reserve reconstructive option if this flap fails?

The rhomboid flap

Small local flaps are frequently employed on the face after the excision of skin lesions. If the defect cannot be closed directly with ease, there may be available a local flap that will produce a better cosmetic result than a graft. However, the most important consideration before using such a flap rather than a graft is a high level of confidence that any malignancy has been completely excised.

The rhomboid (or Limberg) flap is very versatile. It is a type of transposition flap with specific geometry allowing optimal arrangement of available skin, and is particularly appropriate to the temple, cheek and neck areas.

Planning

The rhomboid flap is transferred by a combination of transposition and advancement. Both the excisional defect and the flap are 60° rhomboids and are made identical in size and shape (Fig. 9.8).

All sides are of equal length and are also equal to the short axis of the rhomboid. For any one rhomboid-shaped defect there are four possible rhomboid flaps available to fill it (Fig. 9.8(c)). When planning the flap, aim to raise it from an area of relatively lax skin and to close

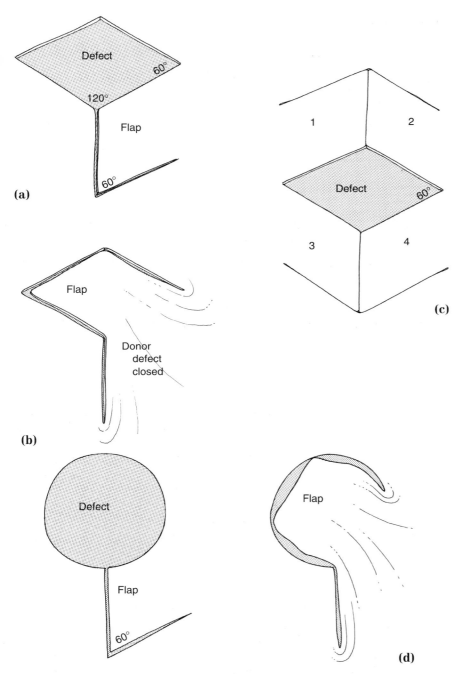

Fig. 9.8 The rhomboid flap: **(a)** Flap design. **(b)** Transposition completed. **(c)** Four available rhomboid flaps. **(d)** Square peg into round hole: (above) flap design; (below) transposition completed.

the donor defect directly and in the line of the skin creases (relaxed skin tension lines). Having determined these two aspects, map out the 'best fit' plan on the skin, after ensuring that adequate tumour clearance is obtained. It is not essential to be precise with the angles; one is operating on skin, which is a mobile and elastic tissue. Indeed it is possible and frequently preferable to excise the lesion in a circular or oval outline and yet still use a rhomboid flap to repair the defect. You can trim the corners of the flap to fit, and the result is a softening of the otherwise sharp angles of the final scars (Fig. 9.8(d)).

Technique

Infiltrate widely beneath both the lesion and the flap with lignocaine and adrenaline, whether or not the patient is under general anaesthesia.

Excise the lesion with a generous layer of underlying fat, and send it for histology. Obtain preliminary haemostasis with bipolar diathermy. After incising its margins, raise the flap with a thickness equivalent to the specimen just removed. Use a skin hook, which is less traumatic than dissecting forceps. The flap has a random pattern vascular supply which is in the subdermal plexus; protect this by raising subcutaneous fat with the flap. Undermine all margins so that easy flap movement and closure are obtained, and then secure haemostasis.

Before suturing the flap in position, close the triangular donor defect where the flap has been raised. Use fine (4/0 or 5/0) Vicryl inverted dermal sutures for this and then tack the flap into place using the same technique. This will hold the skin in the new position and remove almost all tension from the skin sutures, which are now inserted using interrupted 5/0 or 6/0 polybutester.

No dressings are required unless you wish to cover the suture lines with 12 mm wide adhesive paper tape. Instruct the patient to rest at home for 48 hours and to avoid stooping and lifting. The sutures should be removed after 5–6 days.

The Z-plasty

The Z-plasty is a manoeuvre for reorienting a scar or line of skin tension by the mutual transposition of two equal triangular skin flaps. It has wide application, particularly in the management of scars or in preventing scar contracture.

Applications

The Z-plasty is useful for the management of scars, for preventing contractures and to reduce or eliminate a web:

- **to relax a linear contracture**: loose available skin is 'borrowed' from each side of the scar and brought across its line producing lengthening;
- **to disguise the line of a scar**: small zigzag interruptions in the line may make a prominent scar less apparent to the eye;
- **to alter the line of a scar**: a scar may be reoriented into a more natural skin line;
- a Z-plasty may be introduced into the primary closure of a linear wound if there is **a risk of longitudinal scar contracture at that site**, e.g. a scar running across a flexion crease;
- **normal or abnormal anatomical webs** on the hand, face or neck are sometimes suitable for elimination or deepening by Z-plasty.

Design

Make the scar to be manipulated the central limb of the Z (Fig. 9.9).

Draw the two outer limbs at equal angles to the central limb, and make all three the same length. The angles are conventionally 60°,

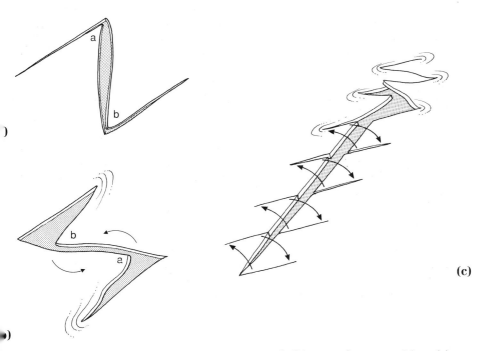

Fig. 9.9   The Z-plasty. **(a)** Design: scar excised. **(b)** Mutual transposition. **(c)** Multiple Z-plasties to release a long scar.

but may be any angle between 30° and 90°. The larger the angle, the greater is the lengthening that will be gained, but the lesser will be the readiness of the flaps to set easily into their new positions.

Where the length of the scar is great in relation to the availability of skin on each side, make a series of multiple Zs (Fig. 9.9(c)). This applies particularly to scar revision on the face, where Z-plasty in any case must be used judiciously and with great caution.

In theory the lengthening produced by a 60° Z-plasty is 75%, or a ratio of 7:4. In reality, cutaneous and subcutaneous scarring, the direction of relaxed skin tension lines and local skin contours all have an influence on the redistribution of the skin involved.

Technique for relaxing a linear scar contracture   Take time to consider and map the lines of incision. It is usual to excise the scar forming the central limb. The angles of the Z need not be exactly 60°. Decide, as the proposed transposition is visualized, which way round the two side arms should be placed so that the flaps move most easily into their new positions and lie as closely as possible to the lines of relaxed skin tension. Do not hesitate to erase the plan and start again. Use multiple Zs if it seems more appropriate. The apex of each triangular flap should be rounded off to avoid necrosis of the tip.

Infiltrate the area with local anaesthetic containing adrenaline.

Excise the scar on the central limb. Incise the other two limbs, outlining the flaps. Raise the two triangular flaps through the subcutaneous fat and make them thicker towards their bases to protect the blood supply. A common cause of partial flap necrosis is making the flap too thin, particularly when operating in areas of scarred skin. Use skin hooks when raising the flaps and undermine the area around their bases, to permit easy transposition.

Place a few inverted 3/0 or 4/0 Vicryl dermal sutures at key points to hold the flaps in their new positions and eliminate tension on the skin sutures. Insert the skin sutures with close, regular spacing taking small bites and just approximating the wound edges. At the apices use a three-point suture (Fig. 9.10) passing transversely

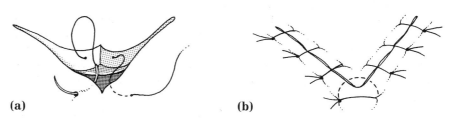

(a)   (b)

Fig. 9.10   The three-point suture. **(a)** Suture placed. **(b)** Wound closed.

through the point of the triangle and emerging to be tied on the surface. This may reduce the risk of flap tip necrosis. Skin tapes may be applied in strategic positions to further reduce tension across the wound margins.

THE INITIAL MANAGEMENT OF MAJOR BURNS

A burn injury is classed as major if its area exceeds 10% of the body surface area in a child or 15% in an adult. These are best managed in a dedicated burns unit, but there may be circumstances where transfer to such a unit is not possible or is significantly delayed. It is important to have a grasp of the principles governing the early treatment of these injuries at such times. In addition, you may have to assess the burn and begin treatment in most cases before the specialized burns team is involved, and the early minutes may be critical to an eventual successful outcome.

Assessment

A serious burn is a form of major trauma and should be managed as such from the outset. Not uncommonly there are concomitant injuries caused either in the accident itself, as in explosions or road accidents, or in the escape from a fire. Do not allow the dramatic appearance of the burn to distract you from considering life-threatening injuries to the head, chest or abdomen. An accurate history of the event is very important.

Attention to the airway and mechanical ventilation may be necessary immediately in cases of blast injury or blunt chest trauma or in severe respiratory injury caused by inhalation of toxic products or hot gases. Look for evidence for an inhalation injury early, as respiratory compromise may develop insidiously. Pointers to note are a history of the fire occurring in an enclosed space such as a building or vehicle and particularly if the victim was trapped. Signs of a possible upper respiratory injury are singeing of facial or nasal hair, facial flame burns, soot on the tongue or pharynx, reddening or swelling of the pharynx, and hoarseness. Any of these should lead to a high level of suspicion; you should then request the following baseline investigations: chest X-ray, arterial blood gases and carboxyhaemoglobin (CoHb) level.

Next assess the patient for associated injuries; these may require urgent intervention before attention is turned to the burn itself. If it is obvious that the burn is extensive, insert an intravenous line in a safe vein with a large cannula and start an infusion of colloid before assessing the burn in detail. Take blood at this time for baseline measurements of haemoglobin, haematocrit, urea and electrolytes, and CoHb if indicated. Achieve analgesia by giving diluted morphine by slow intravenous injection, titrating the volume against pain. Insert a urinary catheter and start a record of output.

Now make a careful examination of the burn, ensuring that you see all areas of the skin. A preliminary assessment can be made in the adult using the Rule of 9s (Fig. 9.11) to judge the total percentage of body surface area burned.

However, this is not accurate in children who have different proportions according to their age. Map out the burn definitively on a printed Lund and Browder chart (Fig. 9.12) and calculate the percentage area.

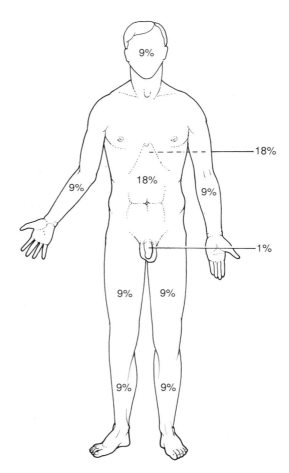

Fig. 9.11 The rule of 9s.

CHART FOR ESTIMATING SEVERITY OF BURN WOUND

NAME_____WARD_____NUMBER_____DATE_____
AGE_____ ADMISSION WEIGHT_____

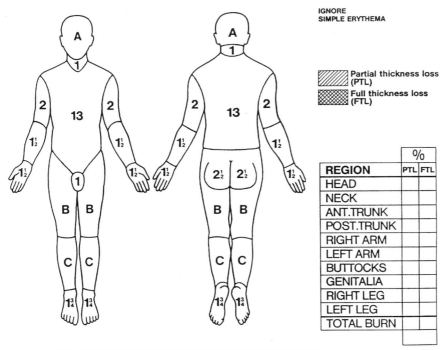

IGNORE
SIMPLE ERYTHEMA

▨ Partial thickness loss (PTL)

▩ Full thickness loss (FTL)

REGION	PTL	FTL
HEAD		
NECK		
ANT.TRUNK		
POST.TRUNK		
RIGHT ARM		
LEFT ARM		
BUTTOCKS		
GENITALIA		
RIGHT LEG		
LEFT LEG		
TOTAL BURN		

RELATIVE PERCENTAGE OF BODY SURFACE AREA AFFECTED BY GROWTH

AREA	AGE 0	1	5	10	15	ADULT
A=½ OF HEAD	9½	8½	6½	5½	4½	3½
B=½ OF ONE THIGH	2¾	3¼	4	4½	4½	4¾
C=½ OF ONE LEG	2½	2½	2¾	3	3¼	3½

Fig. 9.12 A Lund and Browder chart. (Source: reproduced by courtesy of Smith & Nephew Pharmaceutical.)

This figure is important and it is worth taking some time to make sure that an accurate recording and calculation have been made. Ignore areas which are erythema only, without swelling or blistering of the skin.

Some indication of the depth of burn in various areas is useful but this may be difficult to assess accurately in the early stages. Painful, moist, red areas are likely to be partial-thickness injuries, while a dry, white or brown leathery appearance is full-thickness. There are many presentations between these two extremes, however, and it should be emphasized that the depth of burn does not influence calculation of intravenous resuscitation requirements.

Resuscitation

Respiratory

Indications for early intubation and ventilation on the intensive care unit include cutaneous burns of the face and neck causing rapidly accumulating oedema, severe carbon monoxide poisoning and chemical damage to the airways caused by inhalation of smoke and toxic gases. Endotracheal intubation, through the nasal route if possible, is preferable to tracheostomy, which has a high infection risk in burned patients. Lesser degrees of respiratory injury may be managed by humidified oxygen, bronchodilators and chest physiotherapy, but the threshold should be low for transfer to the ICU or suitably equipped burns unit. Flexible bronchoscopy should be resorted to early for both diagnostic and therapeutic indications.

Circulatory

A very large fluid loss occurs from the intravascular compartment over the first 48 hours following a major burn injury. This loss approximates to plasma and gives rise in untreated cases to 'burns shock'. The object of resuscitation is to keep pace with and correct the loss, which often requires many litres of intravenous solution over the initial few hours.

In the UK, resuscitation fluid is usually given in the form of colloid (crystalloid in the USA) as human albumin solution (HAS). The volumes required are maximal in the first 12 hours and gradually reduce over the subsequent 2 days. The Muir and Barclay formula is used to calculate requirements and gives a volume for each of six time-periods in the first 36 hours, the periods comprising 4, 4, 4, 6, 6 and 12 hours respectively. Calculate the volume by multiplying the percentage body surface area burned (BSA) by half the body weight in kilograms, i.e. volume (in ml) = %BSA × weight in kg/2. It is therefore important to have an accurate estimation of the percentage burn, and also to weigh the patient at an early opportunity.

Having made the calculation, adjust the infusion of HAS to run at a rate giving that volume in the first 4-hour period. Measure the period from the time of the burn and not from any subsequent point. This will entail catching up with time lost before the infusion was set up so that the correct volume is given by the end of 4 hours.

A benefit of dividing the resuscitation time into six periods is in having a periodic reminder to reassess the patient's status before prescribing fluid for the next period. The calculated volume is merely a guideline and must be adjusted upwards or downwards if indicated by monitoring, the most important parameter being the hourly urine output. The end of the resuscitation phase using the Muir and Barclay regime is reached after 36 hours, but some fluid loss continues after this time and it is wise to continue some infusion of colloid until at least 48 hours have elapsed.

Insensible water loss requires replacement by the most appropriate route; the frequency of nausea and vomiting in the first two days after a major burn means that an intravenous infusion is often indicated. A solution such as 5% dextrose may be given in parallel with the main resuscitation fluid.

Intravenous resuscitation in this manner should proceed to its conclusion without significant problems as long as the patient is carefully monitored throughout. Exceptions may occur in patients already compromised in their cardiac or renal function or in those with extensive deep burns where high circulating levels of haemoglobin and muscle pigments may cause renal failure.

Monitoring

Because of the large volumes of fluid being exchanged, close monitoring of the patient's resuscitation status is mandatory. In addition to the vital signs, a very useful parameter is the temperature gradient between core and periphery. A difference of 3–4°C indicates satisfactory volume replacement in an otherwise stable subject.

Record the urine output hourly and maintain it at least 0.5 ml per kilogram body weight in each hour, or 10 ml per hour in small children. If volumes fall below these levels for two consecutive hours, check the catheter to ensure that it is patent and in the bladder, and then give a bolus of intravenous fluid and observe the effect.

Further monitoring requires periodic assessments of haematocrit and urine osmolality. Avoid central venous pressure lines and other invasive monitoring techniques because of the increased risks of septicaemia, unless there are serious renal or myocardial complications.

General support

Do not give antibiotics routinely as prophylaxis except in children under the age of 10 who may be given flucloxacillin for the first 5 days to reduce the risk of toxic shock syndrome. Otherwise, reserve systemic antibiotics for specific therapeutic indications as they arise.

For dressings use simple, well-padded paraffin gauze, until the team responsible for surgical management have reviewed the burn. Leave areas on the face and genitalia exposed. Burns that are clearly full-thickness and awaiting excision and grafting may be dressed with silver sulphadiazine cream, but this will heavily disguise the appearance of the burn and make diagnosis of depth difficult; it should be avoided until the responsible surgeon has seen the injuries. The same rule applies to hand burns, which may then be thickly spread with silver sulphadiazine cream and elevated in polythene bags that are changed daily. Other dressings should be changed every 2–3 days, depending on depth of burn, type of dressing and amount of exudate. Dressing changes on larger burns should be done under a general anaesthetic, which also gives opportunity for the physiotherapist to put all affected joints through a full range of passive movement.

It is important to pay careful attention to pain relief and the assistance of a specialist pain-control team is invaluable. Finally, specialist support may also be required from the clinical psychologist, although informal help in this direction should be constantly available from all of the patient's carers.

Cardiothoracic surgery

10

David Weeden and Victor T. Tsang

This chapter outlines the operative techniques that a basic surgical trainee may be called upon to perform in thoracic and cardiac surgery.

BASIC THORACIC SURGICAL TECHNIQUES

Bedside procedures

Chest aspiration

Aspiration of a pleural effusion may be required for diagnostic or therapeutic purposes.

Position   Position the patient sitting on the edge of the bed, leaning slightly forwards with the forearms resting on a stable bed table for support. Use a fine needle to infiltrate the chest wall with local anaesthetic in either the fifth or sixth intercostal space about 3 cm lateral to erector spinae, which will be just below and medial to the inferior pole of the scapula. Aim to pass over the upper border of the rib, to avoid damaging the neurovascular bundle. Unless there is gross pleural thickening the distance between the rib and the pleural space is 5–10 mm.

Procedure   Aspirate an adequate volume of fluid for microbiological culture and cytology using a fine-bore needle. Aspiration of a large volume or of viscous fluid requires the insertion of a wider-bore needle. Chest aspiration sets usually contain appropriate needles, lengths of plastic tubing, a 20 and 50 ml syringe and a three-way tap. Position the needle just within the pleural cavity and grip it, at skin level, with a small artery forceps to prevent excessive movement of the needle, which may damage the lung. Separate the needle from the three-way tap with a length of plastic tubing to allow manipulation of the tap without disturbing the needle position (Fig. 10.1). Take care to prevent air entering the pleural space.

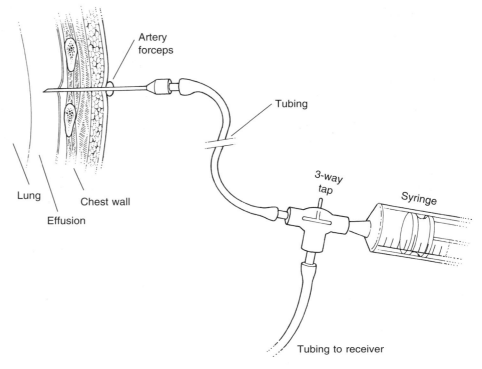

Fig. 10.1   Aspiration of the chest.

Steady withdrawal of fluid leads to expansion of the lung, which may result in the patient coughing. Withdraw the needle when fluid enters the syringe in a jerky fashion and more easily on expiration, or when coughing becomes more frequent. Failure of the lung to expand during aspiration results in a tight feeling in the chest: stop aspiration at this point. The danger of pulmonary oedema from aspiration of large volumes of fluid is exaggerated but volumes in excess of 1500 ml are best drained slowly and completely by insertion of an intercostal drain.

Complications of chest aspiration

- Bleeding from damage to the neurovascular bundle;
- Excessive mediastinal shift when the lung is unable to expand;
- Damage to the lung leading to air leakage;
- Re-expansion pulmonary oedema;
- Damage to abdominal organs by aspiration too low in the chest.

Intercostal drainage

Insert an intercostal drain between the anterior and midaxillary lines above the fifth rib. Use a 24 French drain for air and a 28 French drain for blood to prevent blockage of the drain by clot. Fully abduct the arm to widen the intercostal space. Infiltrate the chest wall with 50 ml of 0.4% lignocaine. Make a 3 cm skin incision over the sixth rib and develop an upwards track with a blunt clip to pass over the top of the fifth rib. The parietal pleura is very sensitive and difficult to infiltrate with local anaesthetic.

> Insert the needle until you aspirate air and withdraw it slowly until the air bubbles stop. Then inject 2–3 ml to anaesthetize the pleura. Warn the patient that there will be 20 seconds of discomfort when the pleura is opened.

Introduce a finger along the track and through the pleura. Sweep it around to confirm that the pleural space has been entered. Insert a simple No. 2 nylon suture where the drain will pass through the incision. Do not use a purse-string suture around the drain as this causes skin necrosis. This suture will be tied when the drain is removed.

Pass the drain through the track into the pleural space with the trocar pulled back 1 cm so the sharp point of the trocar is shielded within the drain. Use the rigidity of the trocar to guide the drain to the desired position (apex for air; posteriorly at the level of the drain site for blood: when the patient is lying semi-recumbent, the lowest part of the hemithorax is the paravertebral area between the sixth and eighth ribs). Fix the drain with a simple No. 2 nylon suture and close the remainder of the wound with interrupted 2/0 nylon sutures.

Occasionally a drain will have to be inserted into a specific area of the chest to drain a loculated collection of air or fluid. The two commonest sites for this are anteriorly in the second intercostal space in the midclavicular line or apically between the first and second ribs through the upper fibres of trapezius. Some loculated collections are best drained under radiological control.

The general management of chest drains is outlined on page 222.

Complications of intercostal drainage

- Bleeding from damage to the neurovascular bundle;
- Damage to the lung;
- Incorrect position of the drain.

Chemical pleurodesis

See page 223.

Endoscopic procedures

Bronchoscopy

Bronchoscopy can be performed with a flexible fibreoptic or a rigid bronchoscope (Table 10.1).

The flexible scope can be passed through the rigid scope. Bronchoscopy requires a good knowledge of bronchial anatomy.

Rigid bronchoscopy   Choose the appropriate size of scope. Place the patient supine and, following induction of general anaesthesia and muscle relaxation, raise the head about 5 cm on a firm pillow with slight extension of the neck. Stand above the head facing the patient's feet and control the maxilla with the middle and ring fingers of your left hand. Hold the scope in your right hand, with the beak positioned anteriorly, and use the thumb and index finger of the left hand to control the scope and protect the upper teeth. Under direct vision, advance the scope in the midline past the uvula, without damaging the lips or tongue, to identify the epiglottis (Fig. 10.2(a)).

Table 10.1   Features of flexible and rigid bronchoscopes

Flexible	*Rigid*
Passed under local anaesthetic	Requires a general anaesthetic
Wider angle of view, superior optics and direct view from distal end of scope	Distal end-viewing and angulated view obtained with with special rigid telescopes
Passes further into bronchial tree to sample more peripheral lesions, especially when performed under X-ray control	Often difficult to visualize beyond segmental bronchi
Can be used in patients with limited cervical movement	Limitation of cervical movement is a contraindication
Difficult to aspirate copious or tenacious sputum or significant quantities of blood	Wide-bore sucker allows easier clearance of secretions and blood
Small size of forceps limits size of biopsy	Large size of forceps allows generous biopsy
Difficult to remove foreign bodies	Easier to remove foreign bodies
Difficult to estimate degree of stenosis or mobility of tracheobronchial tree	Easier to estimate degree of stenosis or mobility of tracheobronchial tree

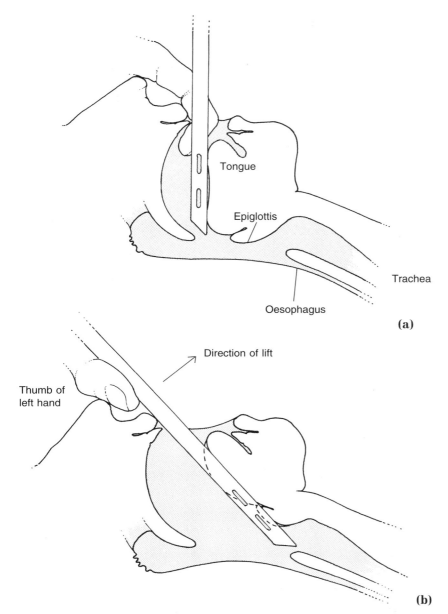

Tongue

Epiglottis

Trachea

Oesophagus

(a)

Direction of lift

Thumb of
left hand

(b)

Fig. 10.2   Insertion of the bronchoscope.

Pass the tip of the scope posterior to the epiglottis then lift it forwards with the thumb and index finger of the left hand while bringing it into a more horizontal position with the right hand (Fig. 10.2(b)). This manoeuvre will displace the tongue and mandible

When laryngeal visualization is poor use a laryngoscope to expose the vocal cords.

anteriorly to allow visualization of the vocal cords. Do not use the upper teeth as a fulcrum for the scope.

If you need to assess the mobility of the vocal cords do not induce muscle relaxation until after the cords have been checked.

Rotate the scope through 90° so that the beak lies in the same axis as the vocal cords, gently pass it through the cords and rotate the scope back to its original position. The scope will normally lie in the right side of the mouth.

Identify the tracheal rings before commencing ventilation with the Sander's injector. Pass the scope into the distal tracheobronchial tree while further extending the neck and rotating the head away from the side being inspected.

Precautions

- Bleeding produced by biopsy must have settled and you must clear the blood from the bronchial tree before the scope is withdrawn.
- Foreign bodies that do not easily fit into the scope should be grasped in appropriate forceps, held in the mouth of the scope and the scope, grasping forceps and foreign body withdrawn together.
- Following removal of a foreign body perform a further full visualization of the tracheobronchial tree.

Flexible bronchoscopy   Adequate nasal, laryngeal and tracheal local anaesthesia is required to allow the transnasal insertion of the flexible bronchoscope. Usually intravenous sedation is required. The technique of transnasal bronchoscopy must be learnt from an experienced bronchoscopist.

Postbronchoscopy position   During recovery from general anaesthesia after bronchoscopy position the patient with the side of the biopsy downwards.

Complications of bronchoscopy

- Bleeding;
- Hypoxia;
- Pneumothorax after transbronchial biopsy;
- Laryngeal oedema in children.

Oesophagoscopy, oesophageal dilatation and intubation

Oesophagoscopy can be performed with a flexible fibreoptic or a rigid scope (Table 10.2).

The flexible scope can be passed through the rigid scope. A barium

Table 10.2 Features of flexible and rigid oesophagoscopes

Flexible	*Rigid*
Passed under local anaesthetic	Requires a general anaesthetic
Wider angle of view, superior optics and direct view from distal end of scope	Distal end-viewing obtained with special rigid telescope
Can be used in patients with limited cervical movement	Limitation of cervical movement is a contraindication
Difficult to enter upper oesophagus in presence of pharyngeal pouch or cricopharyngeal spasm	Easier to enter upper oesophagus in presence of pharyngeal pouch or cricopharyngeal spasm
Difficult to visualize and biopsy lesions in the upper oesophagus	Easier to visualize and biopsy lesions in the upper oesophagus
Can visualize oesophagogastric junction from below, stomach and duodenum	Difficult to pass beyond lower third of oesophagus
Fine flexible scope may pass through strictures	Large size and rigidity precludes passage through strictures
Small size of forceps limits size of biopsy	Large size of forceps allows generous biopsy
Difficult to clear food debris in obstructed oesophagus	Easier to clear food debris in obstructed oesophagus
Difficult to remove foreign bodies	Easier to remove foreign bodies

swallow is advisable before oesophagoscopy in patients with significant dysphagia.

Rigid oesophagoscopy   Choose the appropriate size of scope (16 mm for an adult woman and 20 mm for an adult man). Lesions in the upper oesophagus are best visualized with a short scope. Place the patient supine and, after induction of general anaesthesia, muscle relaxation and endotracheal intubation, moderately extend the neck. Stand above the head facing the patient's feet. Hold the scope in the right hand. Grip the maxilla using the fingers of the left hand, with the thumb along the upper lip to protect the lip and upper teeth. Under direct vision advance the scope in the midline past the uvula, without damaging the lips or tongue (Fig. 10.3(a)), and lift the tongue forward using the thumb of the left hand as a fulcrum for the scope (Fig. 10.3(b)).

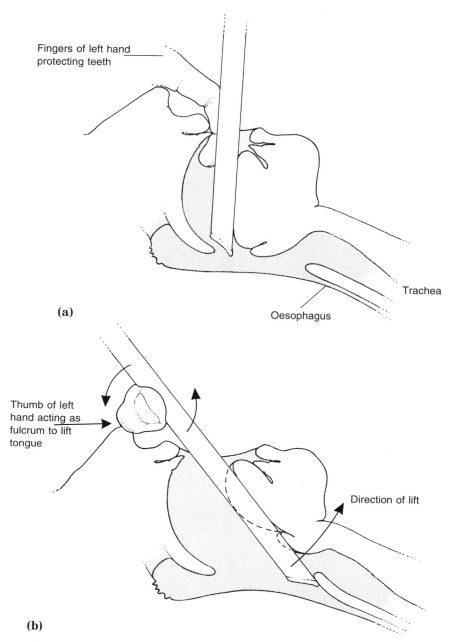

Fingers of left hand
protecting teeth

Trachea

Oesophagus

(a)

Thumb of left
hand acting as
fulcrum to lift
tongue

Direction of lift

(b)

Fig. 10.3   Insertion of the oesophagoscope.

Pass the scope through the cricopharyngeus muscle without force. If cricopharyngeus will not relax with gentle pressure from the beak of the scope, withdraw the scope, visualize cricopharyngeus using a laryngoscope and pass a 50 French Maloney bougie through cricopharyngeus, and then reinsert the scope. If cricopharyngeus still fails to relax, pass a 28 French Maloney bougie through cricopharyngeus and use the bougie as a guide for the scope, remembering that the bougie prevents visualization during passage of the scope and increases the risk of mucosal damage.

Extend the neck as the scope is gently passed down the oesophagus under direct vision. Take great care in passing the scope beyond the mid-third of the oesophagus, about 30 cm from the incisor teeth, as the distal third of the oesophagus curves forwards and the neck cannot usually be extended sufficiently to maintain the straight line that is required to advance the scope. Record the distance from the upper teeth to the lesion, using the centimetre scale on the scope.

Flexible oesophagoscopy   An end-viewing scope is required for oesophagoscopy. If there is resistance to the passage of the scope through cricopharyngeus use a laryngoscope to elevate the larynx and pass the tip of the scope through cricopharyngeus under direct vision. If this fails, gently pass a Maloney bougie under direct vision. Use extreme care when inserting a flexible scope in a patient with a pharyngeal pouch.

Oesophageal dilatation   Following oesophagoscopy, dilate a mild to moderate stricture using Maloney bougies passed through the mouth. Take care when passing small bougies as these may fail to enter the stricture and curl back up the oesophagus. Dilate severe strictures with small Maloney bougies passed through the rigid scope or use a guide wire and coaxial dilators, for example Keymed Advanced Dilators. Difficult strictures are best dilated under X-ray control. Eccentric or rigid strictures may resist the forward pressure of the dilator and can be dilated using a dilating balloon passed over a guide wire. Aim to dilate to 60 French (about 20 mm diameter). Rigid strictures require a smaller initial dilatation with subsequent dilatations to reach 60 French.

Oesophageal intubation   Oesophageal intubation can be achieved by endoscopic pulsion with a rigid tubular stent, which is effective and relatively low-cost, or with an expanding metal stent, which gives slightly superior swallowing and can be inserted higher in the oesophagus without disturbing laryngeal function, but is expensive, or by traction *via* a laparotomy.

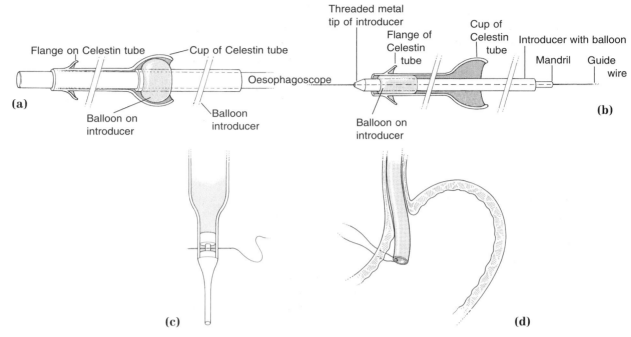

Fig. 10.4 **(a)** Pulsion intubation over flexible oesophagoscope. **(b)** Pulsion intubation over guide wire. **(c)** Connection of traction Celestin tube to pilot bougie. **(d)** Fixation of traction Celestin tube.

Pulsion intubation Dilate the tumour to 60 French, measure the length of the tumour using a flexible scope so the shortest tube length can be used. Place the correct length Medoc Pulsion Celestin tube on the tube introducer, which grips the funnel of the tube by inflation of the balloon on the end of the introducer (Fig. 10.4(a)).

Lubricate the inside and outside of the tube and introducer then thread the scope through the introducer and tube. Reinsert the scope through the tumour and advance the tube over the scope. There will be some resistance to the passage of the tube through the tumour, which becomes greater as the funnel of the tube impacts in the tumour. Use the scope to check that the lower end of the tube has passed beyond the tumour. Deflate the balloon on the introducer and partially withdraw the introducer to confirm the correct position of the top of the tube above the tumour.

When the dilatation or tube placement is difficult carry out the procedure under X-ray control using a guide wire and Medoc mandrel set. Introduce a guide wire and dilate the tumour. Use the scope to measure the length of the tumour and mark the position of the tumour on the X-ray monitor. Place the correct length Medoc Pulsion Celestin tube on the assembled mandrel set (Fig. 10.4(b)), inflate the balloon to grip the tube, lubricate the outside of the tube and the inside of the tube above the balloon, but not at the level of the balloon or it will not grip the tube adequately. Pass the tube and mandrel over the guide wire and confirm the correct tube position radiologically. The flange on the lower end of the tube springs open when it has passed beyond the tumour. Deflate the balloon on the mandrel, gently twist the mandrel to release it from the tube and withdraw the mandrel without displacing the tube. Pass the scope to confirm correct tube placement.

Traction intubation   Use the rigid scope to measure the distance from the incisors to the top of the tumour and pass the pilot bougie of the Traction Celestin tube through the tumour to the stomach. Secure the tube to the end of the pilot bougie with a strong suture (Fig. 10.4(c)). Perform an upper midline laparotomy, pick up the anterior wall of the stomach with Babcock forceps as close to the oesophagogastric junction as possible and insert two 2/0 polyglactin stay sutures. Using diathermy, open the anterior wall of the stomach between the stay sutures. Complete sterility is impossible, but try to minimize contamination. Retrieve the end of the pilot bougie and pull the bougie and tube through the tumour till the cup of the tube is impacted in the tumour. The distance measurements on the tube relate to the previously measured distance from the incisors to the top of the tumour and serve a guide to the correct position of the tube. Cut the lower end of the tube 2 cm below the tumour or as close to the oesophagogastric junction as possible. Pass a No. 2 nylon suture through the wall of the stomach close to the lesser curve, in and out through the tube near its cut end, back through the wall of the stomach and tie it over a piece of greater omentum (Fig. 10.4(d)).

   If the pilot bougie cannot be passed from above either pass a guide wire into the stomach under radiological control and use this to pull the pilot bougie into the stomach or carry out retrograde dilatation through the gastrotomy using a small Maloney bougie and use this to pull the pilot bougie into the stomach. Close the gastrotomy in two layers and use a standard laparotomy closure.

Post-procedure observation   Routine cervical and chest X-rays are required if difficulty was experienced during dilatation. A penetrated chest X-ray is required to confirm the position of the tube after intubation. Recommence oral intake as soon as the effects of the anaesthetic have worn off or bowel sounds have returned after traction intubation. When the tube crosses the oesophagogastric junction there will be free reflux of gastric content into the oesophagus. Tachycardia, fever, surgical emphysema in the neck or pain on swallowing suggest a perforation and an immediate water-soluble contrast swallow is required. If no leak is seen, obtain a barium swallow as water-soluble swallows miss about 30% of small perforations.

Complications of oesophagoscopy, dilatation and intubation

- Aspiration of oesophageal contents during induction of anaesthesia.
- Perforation of the oesophagus above a stricture.
- Splitting of a stricture during dilatation or intubation.
- Too short a tube failing to relieve the obstruction.
- Too long a tube increasing resistance to the passage of food.
- Obstruction of the lower end of the tube on the greater curvature.
- Impairment of laryngeal function when the top of the tube is too close to cricopharyngeus.

Procedures in the neck

Tracheostomy

Tracheostomy can be used to treat or prevent sputum retention, to reduce the risk of laryngeal or tracheal damage when endotracheal intubation is required for more than 10 days, to facilitate weaning from mechanical ventilation and to reduce the work of breathing by excluding upper airways resistance. Sputum clearance can be achieved using a mini-tracheostomy whereas the other indications require a normal tracheostomy.

Mini-tracheostomy   Use a Portex Mini-Trach II Seldinger set. Position the patient supine with the head and neck fully extended and stand above the head facing the patient's feet. A very breathless patient may have to sit upright with the neck extended and the head supported on pillows. If you are right-handed, you will find it easiest to stand on the patient's right. Locate, by palpation, the position of the cricothyroid membrane, which lies immediately below the prominence of the thyroid cartilage, and mark this position on the skin. Infiltrate the skin down to the level of the membrane with 2 ml of 1% lignocaine with adrenaline. If the membrane becomes impalpable, massage the area to disperse the lignocaine. Make a vertical incision, 1 cm in length, in the midline over the membrane, using the special guarded scalpel in the set. Stabilize the larynx by gripping it between the thumb and first finger of the left hand. Fit the 16 gauge Tuohy needle on a syringe and insert it through the membrane with the bevel of the needle facing down the trachea. Confirm proper entry into the trachea by aspirating air freely into the syringe. Remove the syringe, inject 2 ml of 1% lignocaine through the needle, pass the guide wire through the needle and then withdraw the needle along the guide wire, without withdrawing the wire. Dilate the tract using the short wide dilator, passed over the guide wire, and withdraw the dilator without withdrawing the wire. Mount the Mini-Trach tube on the curved introducer and insert both into the trachea over the guide wire. Finally, remove the guide wire and introducer. Fix the tube in place using the neck tapes and pass a suction catheter to clear any blood or secretions.

Open tracheostomy   After induction of general anaesthesia, position the patient supine with a sandbag under the shoulders and the head supported on a ring, to fully extend the neck. Make a 4 cm transverse skin incision half way between the cricoid cartilage and sternal notch. Deepen the incision, using diathermy, to the level of the strap muscles. Control any bleeding from anterior jugular veins by ligation with polyglactin ties. Separate the strap muscles in the midline and retract the strap muscles laterally. Divide the pretracheal fascia to expose the upper tracheal rings and retract the thyroid isthmus cranially. On occasions, the thyroid isthmus requires division between ligatures. Place a 2/0 polyglactin suture in the anterior wall of the trachea immediately above the second ring and leave the needle on the suture (Fig. 10.5(a)).

Confirm that an appropriate-sized cuffed plastic tracheostomy tube, with obturator, is available. The tube should be about two-thirds of the diameter of the trachea and is usually 1–2 mm larger in diameter than the endotracheal tube. A range of tube sizes and sterile connections to reach the anaesthetic circuit beyond the sterile field must be available. Ask the anaesthetist to deflate the endotracheal tube cuff and withdraw the tube till the proximal edge of the cuff is just below the level of the vocal cords and then to reinflate the cuff. Stabilize the trachea by applying downwards traction on the tracheal suture, then incise the anterior two-thirds of the membranous trachea with a scalpel below and clear of the first tracheal ring without, if possible, puncturing the cuff of the tube. Extend the lateral ends of the tracheal incision vertically through the second and third rings. Pass the suture through the subcutaneous tissue of the lower edge of the incision and tighten the suture, which exposes the lumen of the trachea. If the endotracheal tube obstructs the tracheostome it can be further withdrawn to allow insertion of the tracheostomy tube.

Withdraw the obturator and connect the tube to the ventilator circuit. Slowly inflate the cuff till the air leak is sealed. Do not fully withdraw the endotracheal tube till the tracheostomy tube is in

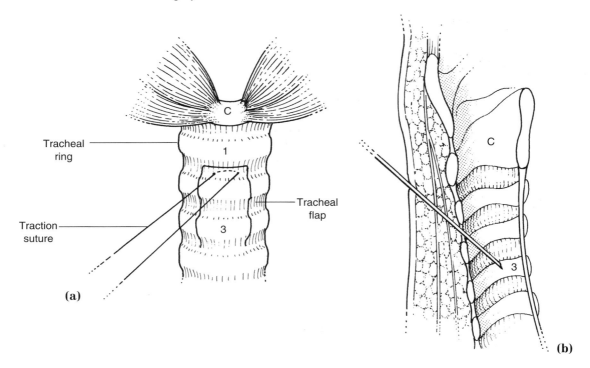

Tracheal ring

Tracheal flap

Traction suture

(a)

C

1

3

C

3

(b)

Fig. 10.5   (a) Open tracheostomy. **(b)** Position of needle puncture during percutaneous tracheostomy. **(c)** Percutaneous tracheostomy guiding catheter. **(d)** Percutaneous tracheostomy dilator.

position and satisfactory ventilation has been established. Using a suction catheter through the tracheostomy tube, clear any blood and retained secretions from the tracheobronchial tree. Ask an assistant to remove the sandbag and, if required, loosely approximate the skin edges with 2/0 colourless polyglactin. Protect the wound with a tracheostomy dressing and stabilize the tube using a neck tape with a Velcro adjustable fastener.

In infants, children and adolescents do not form a tracheal flap but vertically incise the second, third and fourth tracheal rings in the midline to allow insertion of the tube. At all times a patient with a tracheostomy in position must be nursed with spare tubes and tracheal dilating forceps immediately available. After 7 days the insertion track will be reasonably stable. Before this time, changing the tube can be difficult and an experienced operator should be available, although temporary endotracheal intubation can be employed if difficulties are encountered.

Change the tube routinely on or shortly after the seventh day and

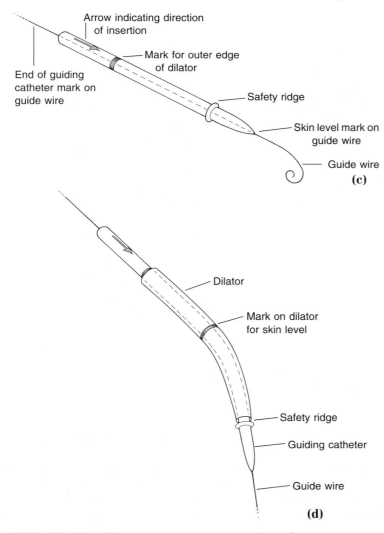

Fig. 10.5   (*Continued*)

thereafter when it becomes encrusted with dried secretions, which make either ventilation or the passage of suction catheters difficult. Clear pharyngeal and tracheal secretions by suction, deflate the cuff and withdraw the tube. Insert the new tube with the tip remaining at right angles to the axis of the trachea till the tip is within the trachea and then rotate the tube so the tip passes down the trachea. Take care to ensure that the tube does not enter the pretracheal space.

Percutaneous dilatational tracheostomy   Percutaneous insertion of a tracheostomy can be carried out using the Ciaglia Introducer set. The technique is contraindicated when the cricoid cartilage is impalpable, if there is significant thyroid enlargement and in children. Position the patient as for an open tracheostomy and withdraw the endotracheal tube so the top of the cuff lies just below the vocal cords. Identify by palpation the thyroid notch and the cricoid cartilage to determine the position of the first and second tracheal rings and mark the skin over the gap between these two rings. Infiltrate the skin and subcutaneous tissues with 4 ml of 1% lignocaine with adrenaline and make a 1.5 cm transverse incision at the point marked between the first and second rings. Using a 19 gauge needle, passed through the skin incision, infiltrate the tissues down to the trachea with a further 4 ml of 1% lignocaine, enter the trachea in the midline, check the position of the needle by confirming free aspiration of air and inject a further 2 ml of lignocaine into the trachea and remove the needle.

Draw up a few millilitres of saline into a syringe attached to the 17 gauge introducing needle and pass this needle through the incision in the midline with the tip angled slightly downwards into the trachea (Fig. 10.5(b)). Aspiration of a steady stream of air bubbles confirms that the trachea has been entered. It is important not to impale the tip of the endotracheal tube. Advance the outer sheath of the introducing needle down the trachea and withdraw the inner needle. Check for free aspiration of air and remove the syringe. Pass the guide wire, J tip foremost, through the sheath and several centimetres into the trachea. Withdraw the sheath without displacing the guide wire and check that the skin level marker on the guide wire is at the level of the incision. Pass the 11 French dilator, which has an integral syringe hub, over the guide wire and into the trachea with a twisting movement, then remove the dilator without withdrawing the guide wire. The 8 French guiding catheter has a safety ridge near the tracheal end and a directional arrow near the other end (Fig. 10.5(c)). Advance the catheter over the guide wire in the direction of the arrow till the tip of the catheter is at the skin level and then advance the catheter and guide wire together till the safety ridge lies at skin level. Check that the distal marker on the guide wire is aligned with the outer end of the guiding catheter.

Position the 12 French blue dilator over the guiding catheter so the tip of the dilator lies against the safety ridge and the outer end of the dilator is aligned with the single marker on the guiding catheter. Advance the guide wire, guiding catheter and dilator together, with a twisting motion, until the skin position mark on the dilator (Fig. 10.5(d)) is at skin level. Pull back and advance the dilator, catheter and guide wire several times without withdrawing the whole assembly further than the safety ridge. Repeat the above dilating procedure with each dilator in turn till the tracheal entry site is dilated to a larger size than the chosen tracheostomy tube (6 mm tube dilate to 24 French, 7 mm to 28 French, 8 mm to 32 French, 9 mm to 36 French), which allows for passage of the tracheostomy balloon.

Test and then totally deflate the cuff on the chosen tracheostomy tube. Lubricate the correct size of dilator and position the tracheostomy tube about 2 cm from the tracheal end of the dilator (6 mm tube over 18 French dilator, 7 mm over 21 French, 8 mm over 24 French, 9 mm over 28 French) then lubricate the outer surface of the tracheostomy tube. Reposition the dilator and tracheostomy tube as during the previous dilatations and advance the tracheostomy tube, dilator, guiding catheter and guide wire together. Once the cuff of the tube is within the trachea withdraw the dilator, guiding catheter and guide wire and advance the tracheostomy tube to its normal position. Inflate the cuff, confirm satisfactory ventilation and remove the endotracheal tube.

The steps in the technique that are particularly important are:

- not to damage the first tracheal ring;
- to confirm proper entry into the trachea by free aspiration of air before placing the guide wire;
- not to impale the tip of the endotracheal tube when initially entering the trachea;
- correct positioning and manipulation of the guide wire, guiding catheter and dilators during dilatation;
- complete deflation of the cuff;
- good lubrication of the tracheostomy tube.

Keep the guide wire, guiding catheter and dilators with the patient in case the tracheostomy tube has to be changed before a tract has formed.

Complications of tracheostomy

- Haemorrhage;
- Tube obstruction (dried secretions, malposition of the tip of the tube allowing impaction against the anterior or posterior wall of the trachea, herniation of an over inflated cuff across the tube tip and displacement of the tube);
- Local infection;
- Tracheal stenosis.

Mediastinal staging procedures

Superior mediastinal nodes can be approached *via* mediastinoscopy but anterior mediastinal nodes or masses can only be reached by anterior mediastinotomy. Superior vena caval obstruction is a relative contraindication to mediastinoscopy because of venous engorgement, although the pretracheal veins are not engorged. An accurate appreciation of the structures surrounding the trachea is required before undertaking mediastinal exploration.

- The innominate vein lies anterior to the trachea.
- The innominate artery lies anterior to and to the right of the trachea.
- The aortic arch and the left common carotid artery lie to the left of the trachea.
- The right pulmonary artery passes anterior to the right main bronchus just caudal to the carina.
- The azygous vein passes postero-anteriorly just above the right tracheobronchial angle.
- The pericardium and left atrium lie inferior to the subcarinal nodes.
- The left recurrent laryngeal nerve runs about 1 cm to the left of the trachea in the midtracheal plane.

Mediastinoscopy Under general anaesthesia, position the patient supine with a sandbag beneath the shoulders, a head ring to stabilize the neck and a slight head-up tilt to lessen venous congestion. Most right-handed operators will find digital mediastinal exploration easiest from the left side of the patient with the endotracheal tube displaced into the right side of the mouth. Make a 4 cm transverse skin incision 1 cm above the suprasternal notch. Deepen the incision, using diathermy, to reach the strap muscles. Separate the strap muscles in the midline. Incise the pretracheal fascia to reach the anterior wall of the trachea. Use the index finger of your right hand to dissect down the anterior wall of the trachea, deep to the pretracheal fascia, then clear both sides of the trachea. Insert the mediastinoscope into the pretracheal space and continue the dissection, using the sucker as a probe, down the anterior aspect of the trachea to the carina, and down the right lateral aspect to the right tracheobronchial angle and the left lateral aspect to the level of the aortic arch. Identify the position of lymph nodes by palpation. Through the mediastinoscope vascular structures look very like nodes, so needle structures to be biopsied with a 21 gauge needle held in long forceps before you take a biopsy. Confirm satisfactory haemostasis. No mediastinal drainage is required. Close the platysma with 2/0 polyglactin and the skin with subcuticular 3/0 polyglactin.

Extended mediastinoscopy It is possible to pass the mediastinoscope between the aortic arch and the left lateral wall of the trachea to reach the left tracheobronchial angle and the subaortic fossa. There is a potential risk of damage to the aortic arch and left recurrent laryngeal nerve and these areas are best approached using a left anterior mediastinotomy.

Anterior mediastinotomy   This approach allows safe biopsy of nodes in the left tracheobronchial angle, the subaortic fossa and masses in the anterior mediastinum not accessible by mediastinoscopy. Make a 5 cm transverse skin incision over the second costal cartilage. Deepen the incision, using diathermy, to reach pectoralis major and split the fibres of the muscle. Open the perichondrium with diathermy, mobilize the costal cartilage subperichondrially, divide the cartilage at the costochondral junction and bend the cartilage outwards and medially to dislocate the chondrosternal junction and remove the cartilage. Avoid the internal mammary artery if possible, but if it is damaged ligate the vascular bundle with 2/0 polyamide in two places and divide the bundle between the ties. Explore the anterior and superior mediastinum digitally and biopsy identified nodes under direct vision. Open the pleura to assess the subaortic fossa. Close pectoralis major with continuous No. 2 polyglactin. If the pleura has been opened ask the anaesthetist to fully expand the lung while you close the last part of pectoralis. No drain is required unless there is an air leak from lung damage.

Complications of mediastinal staging   Bleeding is rare and usually can be controlled by packing the mediastinum with ribbon gauze. If bleeding recurs following removal of the gauze, repack the mediastinum, close the wound and remove the pack after 24 hours. Bleeding sufficient to cause haemodynamic instability requires an exploratory thoracotomy on the appropriate side.

Thoracoscopy

Simple thoracoscopy is used in the investigation of pleural effusions and to create pleurodesis. Video-assisted thoracoscopic surgery (VATS) can be used for some intrathoracic surgical procedures.

Diagnostic thoracoscopy

After induction of general anaesthesia and double-lumen endotracheal intubation, place the patient in the lateral thoracotomy position. If necessary, thoracoscopy can be performed using local anaesthesia with the patient in the semi-lateral position. Use a 19 gauge needle for diagnostic aspiration in the fifth or sixth intercostal space in the midaxillary line to confirm that an effusion is present so the scope can be introduced safely. In a patient with no effusion a pneumothorax can be induced, but this is a potentially difficult technique which must be learnt from an experienced surgeon.

Send a sample of the effusion for cytological and microbiological investigation. Make a 2 cm skin incision at the site of the aspiration and gently introduce the trocar and stylette into the pleural space. Withdraw the stylette and pass a 20 French drain through the trocar. Attach suction tubing to the drain, with a Y connector, and completely drain the effusion, intermittently allowing air to enter the pleural space *via* the open end of the Y connector. Insert the scope through the trocar to visualize the pleural surfaces. Use the integral biopsy forceps to sample the parietal pleura in a number of areas. Superficial biopsies of the visceral pleura can be taken but there is a risk of air leakage.

Withdraw the scope, insert the drain through the trocar and withdraw the trocar. Place a simple No. 2 nylon suture in the midpart of the incision, to be tied when the drain is removed, and anchor the drain with a further No. 2 nylon suture. Do not apply suction to the chest drain till a chest X-ray has confirmed reasonable expansion of the lung. The general management of chest drains is outlined on page 222.

Powder pleurodesis   After diagnostic thoracoscopy, insufflate 20 g of sterile talc or kaolin powder through the trocar. Pleural adhesion will occur only if the visceral and parietal pleura are in apposition.

Complications of thoracoscopy

- Significant bleeding from the biopsy site; this is uncommon and requires insertion of a separate shielded diathermy probe for coagulation.
- Intrapleural infection.
- Air leak from damage to the lung.
- Excessive mediastinal shift from suction on the drain in the presence of a non-expanding lung.

Approaches to intrathoracic structures

The choice of approach to intrathoracic structures depends on the procedure to be performed (Table 10.3).

The commonest approach is a posterolateral thoracotomy, with independent ventilation of the lungs using a double-lumen endobronchial tube, with the endobronchial component passed into the main bronchus of the side opposite that of the planned procedure.

Table 10.3 Approaches to intrathoracic structures

Approach	Indication
Posterolateral	Commonest incision for exposure of one hemithorax
Auscultatory triangle	Apical pleurectomy
Anterior	Emergency relief of cardiac tamponade, open lung biopsy, pericardial window
Posterior	Procedure on grossly infected lung when lung isolation is not possible
Thoracolaparotomy	Exploration of the abdomen and one hemithorax – oesophgogastrectomy, liver trauma
Median sternotomy	Cardiac surgery, simultaneous exposure of both hemithoraces
Midline laparotomy + median sternotomy	Exploration of abdomen + both hemithoraces

Posterolateral thoracotomy

Place the patient in the lateral position after intubation with a double-lumen tube. The lateral position is held using either thoracotomy table supports or a surgical moulding mattress. Make a curved incision starting midway between the medial border of the scapula and the vertebral spines, usually from the level of the fifth rib, to pass 2 cm below the inferior pole of the scapula, curving downwards towards the midaxillary line. Deepen the incision, using diathermy, through the subcutaneous fat to reach latissimus dorsi, and divide this muscle at the lower margin of the wound. There is no need to divide the lower fibres of trapezius in the posterior angle of the wound. Deep to latissimus lies serratus anterior in the anterior half of the wound, with a fascial layer in the posterior half. Divide the fascia behind serratus to expose the ribs. Lift the scapula to count the ribs posteriorly, remembering that it is difficult to feel the first rib, because of the attachment of scalenus posterior. Choose the appropriate rib bed for the exposure required (Table 10.4).

Score the centre line of the chosen rib with the diathermy from the erector spinae muscle to the point at which serratus anterior originates from that rib. Using a periosteal elevator, strip the periosteum from the upper edge of the rib, from posterior to anterior, keeping the handle of the elevator at right angles to the rib so as not to damage the underlying lung.

Table 10.4 Intercostal space used during thoracotomy

Rib bed	Type of operative procedure
4th	Aortic arch, aortic isthmus, innominate and subclavian arteries
5th	Upper or middle lobectomy, apical pleurectomy
6th	Lower lobectomy, pneumonectomy, decortication, exploration for trauma
7th	Oesophagogastrectomy, extended oesophagomyotomy
8th	Antireflux procedures, oesophagomyotomy, repair of ruptured diaphragm

Divide the costotransverse ligament with a notched elevator, to prevent strain injury to the ligament when spreading the ribs. This is preferable to dividing the rib at its posterior angle, which increases traction injury on the intercostal nerve. Removing a rib does not improve exposure. Open the parietal pleura carefully with a scalpel, in case of adhesions. Divide any pleural adhesions around the thoracotomy site by sharp dissection before inserting a mechanical rib spreader and then divide the remaining adhesions to mobilize the lung. If serratus anterior restricts exposure divide it close to its insertion to preserve the nerve supply. Cut the muscle from its posterior edge to the belly arising from the opened intercostal space.

Auscultatory triangle

Place the patient in the lateral position after intubation with a double-lumen tube. Make a 10 cm incision over the auscultatory triangle (bounded medially by the lateral border of the lower fibres of trapezius, laterally by the medial border of the scapula and inferiorly by the upper border of latissimus), parallel to and 2 cm from the medial border of the scapula, starting 1 cm behind the inferior pole of the scapula. Enter the chest through the bed of the fifth rib.

Anterior thoracotomy

Place the patient supine, intubated with a single- or double-lumen tube. Make a 10 cm incision in the interspace below the nipple from the sternal edge towards the axilla, deepen the incision, using diathermy, through pectoralis major to reach the ribs. In an emergency divide pectoralis major with a scalpel. Enter the chest through the bed of the fourth or fifth rib. Insert a mechanical rib spreader. To improve exposure, in emergency situations, divide the anterior costal cartilages above and below the opened space or make a transverse sternal extension.

Posterior thoracotomy

Place the patient prone, intubated with a single-lumen tube, with shoulders and pelvis supported to allow chest expansion. Both main bronchi angle anteriorly forwards from the carina, so in this position they lie below the level of the carina. This position prevents contaminated secretions passing from one lung to the other. Lung isolation is usually obtained with a double-lumen tube but this may not be feasible in small adults and children in whom the posterior approach is valuable. Start the incision more posteriorly than in lateral thoracotomy; otherwise the procedure is the same.

Thoracolaparotomy

Place the patient in the lateral position after intubation with a double-lumen tube. Make a lateral thoracotomy incision and extend the incision anteriorly to cross the costal margin, between the sixth and seventh costal cartilages, for about 5 cm towards the umbilicus. Enter the chest through the bed of the seventh rib, divide the costal margin in this line and resect part of the costal arcade (Fig. 10.6(a)) so that it will not splint the ribs apart during closure.

Additional abdominal exposure can be obtained by extending the incision as a paramedian or midline laparotomy. Open the diaphragm circumferentially, about 2 cm from its origin, over about 10 cm.

Median sternotomy

Place the patient supine, intubated with a single-lumen tube (or use a double-lumen tube if performing a pulmonary procedure). Make a vertical incision from the suprasternal notch to the tip of the xiphisternum. Deepen the incision, using diathermy, to reach the midline of the sternum. Divide the transverse suprasternal ligament so that a finger can be inserted behind the sternum. Free one side of the xiphisternum to allow a finger to be inserted behind the sternum to strip the pleura away from the midline. Divide the sternum, from below upwards, in the midline using a powered vertically oscillating saw. During division of the sternum disconnect the endotracheal tube to deflate the lungs. Use diathermy to control significant periosteal bleeding.

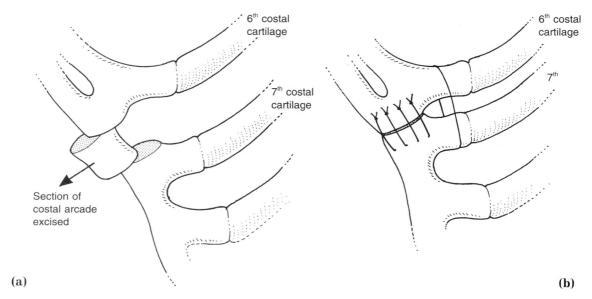

(a)

(b)

Fig. 10.6 **(a)** Costal arcade in thoracolaparotomy incision. **(b)** Suturing of costal arcade after thoracolaparotomy.

Median sternotomy and midline laparotomy

This approach is used for exposure of both hemithoraces and the abdomen. Make a median sternotomy as described above and extend the incision downwards in the midline as far as is required to expose the abdominal cavity.

Placement of drains

Use plastic drains, with multiple side-holes and a radio-opaque marker. In adults use 28 French size to prevent blood clot occluding the drain. Make separate skin stab wounds, below the level of the incision, anterior to the posterior axillary line so the patient does not lie on them, and adequate in length to accommodate the drain without undue skin tension. Place a simple No. 2 nylon suture through the centre of the drain incision and leave it long with the ends knotted, to be tied when the drain is removed. Place a second No. 2 nylon suture at the end of the drain incision to fix the drain. With a swab inside the chest wall, to protect the lung, push a Robert's forceps through the intercostal muscles and draw the drain out from within the chest.

Most intrathoracic procedures require the use of one or two drains, depending on the degree of air leakage and bleeding. If one drain is used, additional side-holes should be cut to allow drainage from the apex to the base. When placing two drains position the posterior drain below the lung to drain fluid (all the Bs – **b**ack, **b**lood, **b**ase) and the anterior drain at the apex (all the As – **a**pex, **a**ir, **a**nterior). Drain a pneumonectomy space with a single low tube. After median sternotomy use a single retrosternal drain brought out through a skin stab in the midline below the incision. If the pleura has been opened, place the end of the drain in the apex of the pleural space and, if both pleural cavities have been entered, use two drains. After thoracolaparotomy, if the opposite mediastinal pleura has been opened, make additional holes in the basal drain and pass the tip of the drain into the opposite pleural cavity through the posterior mediastinum. Use a simple underwater seal bottle to connect to the drain.

Closure of thoracotomy incisions

Close incisions involving intercostal spaces with No. 2 polyglactin sutures, passed over the upper rib and below the lower rib of the space opened, taking care to pass the suture close to the lower edge of the inferior rib so as not to include the intercostal bundle. Hold the ribs together by digital approximation and progressive tightening of the pericostal sutures. Avoid the use of a mechanical rib approximator if possible. Gentle downwards pressure on the shoulder, usually by the anaesthetist, returns the scapula to its normal position and allows the two muscle layers to be closed with a continuous No. 2 polyglactin suture. Use a subcutaneous and subcuticular polyglactin suture to complete the closure. After thoracolaparotomy reapproximate the edges of the diaphragm with a single layer of continuous No. 2 polyglactin, taking good bites but avoiding the branches of the phrenic nerve, suturing from either end of the incision, closing the posterior rectus sheath in the same layer as the diaphragm.

If the costal margin has been divided, reapproximate it with four No. 2 polyglactin sutures (Fig. 10.6(b)) as well as four or six pericostal sutures. After median sternotomy reapproximate the sternum with heavy steel wire, taking care to pass the wires close to the lateral edges of the sternum. Do not overtighten the wires, to prevent them from cutting through the bone. The wires must not be passed lateral to the edges of the sternum or the internal mammary artery may be damaged. Close the remainder of the wound in layers with absorbable sutures.

Postoperative care

Post-thoracotomy analgesia

Intravenous narcotic patient-controlled analgesia (PCA) is very effective.

When the parietal pleura is still present a thin, plastic catheter, e.g. an epidural catheter, can be placed in the extrapleural space to allow a continuous infusion of local anaesthetic, e.g. 6 ml/h of 0.25% bupivacaine. Strip the posterior parietal pleura from the chest wall to form a pouch three ribs above and below the incision. Use a Tuohy needle to pass the catheter through the chest wall into the lowest part of the pouch, placing the tip in the highest part of the pouch.

A continuous thoracic epidural infusion of a narcotic and local anaesthetic mixture provides excellent analgesia but this must be set up by an experienced anaesthetist, who will advise on the appropriate drugs and their doses.

Postoperative management of drains

Apply low-pressure (up to 5 kPa) high-volume suction to most chest drains to encourage early complete expansion of the lung. A Robert's pump should not be used as this produces low-volume suction. Do not apply suction to a pneumonectomy space drain; clamp it and release the clamp for 2 min every 4 hours. This will allow the mediastinum to move slightly towards the operated side, although excessive mediastinal movement should be avoided. In circumstances where the ability of the lung to expand fully is in doubt, increasing suction should be applied slowly to check that there is not excessive mediastinal movement.

Remove a pneumonectomy space drain on the first postoperative day. With two drains *in situ* remove the basal drain when the drainage is below 200 ml/d and there is no air leak through the drain, usually on the first or second postoperative day. Remove a single drain or the apical (second) of a pair of drains when the lung is fully expanded and there has been no air leak for 24 hours. Except when draining a pneumonectomy space, chest drains should not be clamped. A trial period of clamping before removing a drain is only required when there has been a prolonged air leak. If the lung is fully expanded but the air leak persists beyond 4 days discontinue the suction and take an X-ray to confirm continuing full expansion. If there has been collapse of the lung reapply suction. Remove a drain without allowing air to enter the chest. Ask the patient to take a deep breath and hold it at the end of inspiration. Remove the tube quickly and smoothly, and tighten the previously placed suture at once.

Procedures for pleural adhesion

Recurrent pneumothoraces require the formation of adhesions between the two layers of the pleura, which will only work when the two layers lie together.

Chemical pleurodesis

After insertion of a chest drain and administration of a narcotic analgesic instil 20 ml of 1% lignocaine through the drain. Alter the patient's position to disperse the lignocaine throughout the pleural cavity. Wait 5 min and then instil tetracycline (for benign conditions use 10–15 mg/kg body weight; for malignant effusions use 20–30 mg/kg) with a further 10 ml of 1% lignocaine. If there is no or only a mild air leak clamp the drain for 2 hours, alter the patient's position to disperse the tetracycline, then reapply suction for 72 hours before removing the drain. With a more significant air leak, loop the drain tube up so that the highest point of the tube is always 10 cm higher than the highest point of the chest during the 2 hours that the tetracycline is being dispersed around the pleural space.

Powder pleurodesis

See page 216.

Pleural abrasion

Enter the pleural space *via* an auscultatory triangle thoracotomy. Abrade the parietal pleura to the point of capillary haemorrhage with a gauze swab or a nylon scourer. Inspect the visible lung surface, especially the apex of the upper lobe, and exclude any small bullae by ligation (2/0 polyamide), suturing (4/0 polydioxanone) or stapling. Insert a single drain and close routinely.

Pleurectomy

Expose the ribs *via* an auscultatory triangle incision. Mobilize the fifth rib subperiosteally without deflating the lung. Separate the parietal pleura from the chest wall around the margins of the incision before inserting a mechanical retractor. Continue to strip the pleura in the layer of the endothoracic fascia using fingers and then a swab on a Rampley's holder. Keep the lung inflated as this helps to prevent the pleura tearing. Strip the pleura upwards, across the apex of the chest and down the mediastinum to the hilum, taking care not to pick up subpleural nerves or vessels. Strip the pleura anteriorly to close to the internal mammary vessels, posteriorly to the costovertebral recess and inferiorly as far as can be reached. Inspect for a site of air leak and seal this if identified. Insert a single drain and close routinely.

VATS pleurectomy

A parietal pleurectomy can be performed in patients without numerous pleural adhesions using an endoscopic approach. This technique, while not difficult, must be taught by an experienced surgeon.

Intrapleural sepsis

In early intrapleural sepsis there is an infected pleural effusion, which should be completely cleared by insertion of a chest drain, to which suction should be applied. Left undrained, the infected material becomes 'walled off' with a thick layer of granulation tissue to produce an empyema. Initial treatment of an empyema is tube drainage, often requiring CT control for accurate placement, to overcome systemic disturbance from infection, which obviates the need for surgical drainage in the acutely unwell patient. A thick-walled chronic empyema usually requires formal surgical intervention by rib resection or decortication.

Rib resection

After induction of general anaesthesia and insertion of a double-lumen tube, place the patient in the lateral thoracotomy position. Having determined the lowest point of the cavity from the chest X-ray or thoracic CT, use a wide-bore needle to confirm the presence of the empyema cavity by aspiration, usually in the posterior axillary line, above and below the rib chosen for resection. Make a 7 cm skin incision along the line of the chosen rib, centred on the posterior axillary line, and deepen the incision, using diathermy, down to the rib. Repeat the aspiration above and below the rib to confirm that the correct position for resection has been chosen and to establish the thickness of the empyema wall. Score the rib, using diathermy, over 5 cm and use a rougine to strip the periosteum from the rib, from posterior to anterior above the rib and from anterior to posterior below the rib. Take care not to damage the intercostal bundle below the rib. Use a costotome to resect a length of rib equal to the vertical distance between the lower border of the rib above to the upper border of the rib below.

With a scalpel incise the periosteum and empyema cavity wall in the rib bed and remove a piece of the empyema wall for histological examination. Clear all the fibrinous material from the cavity using a sucker and gauze swabs and send a specimen for culture. Insert a red rubber tube drain, of greater than 1.5 cm diameter, about 2 cm into the part of the cavity that will be lowest in the semi-recumbent position. There should be no side-holes in the tube as these allow ingrowth of granulation tissue, which may obstruct the lumen of the tube and make withdrawal of the tube difficult. If the cavity extends down to the diaphragm, place the tube one interspace above the lowest point of the cavity as the diaphragm will rise during the obliteration of the space. The drainage tube usually enters the cavity at or behind the posterior axillary line but the tube should exit through the skin at or in front of the posterior axillary line so that the patient does not have to lie on the exit site, which causes increased pain.

Suture the chest wall muscles with No. 2 polyglactin and the skin with interrupted 2/0 nylon. Fix the drain with a No. 2 nylon suture and connect to an underwater seal, initially without suction. When the drainage reduces to less than 200 ml/d cut the drain about 5 cm beyond the skin, remove the drain fixation suture, transfix the drain with a safety pin without occluding the lumen and fix the tube with narrow strapping to the skin (Fig. 10.7).

Cover the protruding part of the drain with a colostomy bag. The tube must remain in place until the cavity is completely obliterated by granulation tissue and this is best assessed by regular sinograms, performed every 4–6 weeks, to delineate the size of the cavity and the

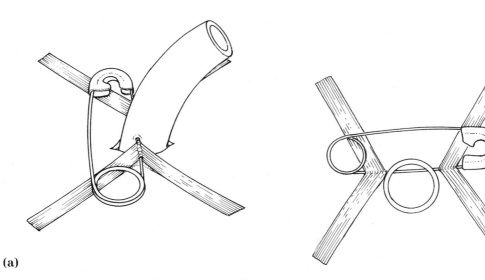

(a)   (b)

Fig. 10.7   Pin and tape fixation for empyema tube.

In the presence of a large bronchopleural fistula rib resection must be performed under local anaesthesia with the patient sitting upright.

dependency of the drain. When no cavity remains the tube can be withdrawn 3 cm to allow progressive healing of the drain track.

Decortication

Decortication involves mobilization of the entire empyema cavity to free the underlying lung. It is a potentially complicated operation and must be supervised by an experienced surgeon.

Emergency cardiac procedures

Survival after penetrating cardiac injury requires tamponade, to temporarily seal the myocardial wound, as free bleeding causes exsanguination.

Pericardiocentesis

The false-positive/negative rate is up to 30%, but pericardiocentesis can produce temporary improvement. Introduce the needle of an 18 gauge Seldinger CVP set to the left of the xiphisternum at 45° to the skin, aiming for the left shoulder, with the V lead of an ECG attached to the needle. When the needle touches the epicardium the QRS complex will invert. If aspiration produces blood, insert the guide wire, then the catheter. Removal of 100–200 ml of blood produces significant improvement in cardiac tamponade, although the improvement may be short-lasting. If there is no improvement the tip of the catheter probably lies within the right ventricle. If immediate exploration of the pericardium is not required, cap off the catheter and leave it in place for 5 days, when adhesions will prevent bleeding on removing the catheter.

Subxiphoid pericardiostomy

This can be used to exclude tamponade in doubtful cases. Induction of general anaesthesia in the presence of cardiac tamponade may lead to a severe fall in blood pressure from vasodilation, so drape the operative site before induction. Make a vertical midline incision over the xiphisternum. Deepen the incision, using diathermy, to reach the xiphisternum and excise it. Behind and slightly above the origin of the xiphisternum is the junction of the anterior pericardium and the diaphragm. Use artery forceps to pick up the pericardium, which in tamponade will be tense and blue, and incise the pericardium with a scalpel. If tamponade is confirmed proceed to a median sternotomy, otherwise close the wound with the tip of a chest drain within the pericardium.

Left anterior thoracotomy

This is the best approach for emergency thoracotomy for penetrating cardiac injury with tamponade. The incision is described on page 218. Open the pericardium longitudinally anterior to the phrenic nerve. The bleeding has often stopped but the site of injury must be identified. Control active bleeding by digital pressure as the myocardial wound is usually small. Control large defects by inserting a spigoted Foley catheter through the defect and inflating the balloon with saline. Do not apply traction to the catheter as this will lead to a worsening myocardial tear. If required, clear the catheter of air and use it for transfusion. Repair myocardial defects with interrupted horizontal mattress 2/0 polypropylene sutures, buttressed with Teflon felt or pericardium. Tighten the sutures so as to just appose the edges of the myocardium, which is very friable. If the myocardial defect lies close to a coronary vessel pass the suture deep to the vessel, to prevent coronary occlusion. Control bleeding from a coronary vessel by passing a 2/0 polypropylene suture deep to the vessel and applying a snugger. A major coronary vessel will require repair but a smaller vessel may be ligated; however, you must obtain expert advice to make this decision. Avoid excessive manipulation of the heart as it reduces output and increases irritability. Full repair of the cardiac injury may require a median sternotomy and cardiopulmonary bypass.

BASIC CARDIAC SURGICAL TECHNIQUES

This section on basic cardiac surgical techniques is intended to provide practical information for you on the cardiac unit. In surgery, attention to detail is essential for the well-being of your patients. Even though your post may be a junior one, try to achieve excellence at all times. You are likely to assist at these procedures many times before you are asked to do them. Each time, mentally talk yourself through the procedure so that you will be ready when your chance comes.

Median sternotomy and cardiopulmonary bypass

Sternotomy

Median sternotomy offers the best approach to the anterior mediastinum, the pericardium and the heart. You must take care to avoid injury to the underlying innominate vein, ascending aorta and right ventricle.

Place the patient in a supine position with the neck slightly extended. Prepare the skin with alcoholic iodine solution. Make a midline incision from the suprasternal notch to the subxiphoid area. With diathermy cut through the subcutaneous tissue, fascia and periosteum of the sternum. Pick up and divide the xiphoid process with cautery. Split the sternum in the midline with either an oscillating or an electric Sarns saw. Cauterize the sternal edges. Occasionally you may need a small amount of bone wax to control bleeding from the marrow. Use a Finochietto retractor to hold the sternal edges apart. Dissect the anterior mediastinal tissue down to the pericardium. Open this in the midline with a diathermy and place silk sutures in each edge to hold them apart.

Dividing the cardiopulmonary bypass circuit

The perfusionist passes up the bypass tubing from the heart–lung bypass machine. Secure them to the drapes. Apply two tubing clamps to the bypass circuit and divide the arterial and venous lines with tubing shears. Make sure that the surgical field is not crowded and keep the lines free of kinks.

Cannulation

For most heart operations performed by median sternotomy, the ascending aorta and the right atrium are cannulated.

Arterial cannulation   Ask the anaesthetist to heparinize the patient and place a concentric purse string (usually 2/0 Ethibond or Ticron) in the distal ascending aorta. Pass the suture through a long, narrow, plastic tube (size 16 French catheter) using an open-eye fine probe. Secure the ends of the purse string suture with a pair of Dunhill artery forceps.

  Ask your assistant to hold a pair of long Roberts forceps to steady the aorta in the left hand, and to have the purse string with its snugger ready in the right hand. Use a No. 11 blade to clear the cannulation site of aortic adventitia, make a stab incision and cover it with a finger. Insert the aortic cannula and ask your assistant to tighten the purse string and snugger over the cannula. Hold it tight by clamping the plastic tube. Tie the snugger to the aortic cannula, which is pointing towards the aortic arch. Connect the aortic cannula to the arterial connection of the circuit with the air bubbles excluded and secure the arterial line to the drape with a silk suture or artery forceps.

Venous cannulation   Place a right atrial purse string (usually 2/0 Ethibond or Ticron) around the atrial appendage and fit a snugger. Apply a side clamp to the appendage. Ask your assistant to hold the side clamp. Incise the tip of the appendage. As the assistant opens the clamp wide, insert the venous cannula through the purse string, and ask your assistant to snug down to secure the cannula. Connect the cannula to the venous line of the bypass circuit *via* a straight connector. Begin bypass as the line clamps are removed. At this stage, the heart is still beating; the patient will be gently cooled.

Coming off bypass and closure of sternotomy

Once the surgical repair is completed, the patient is rewarmed back to normal temperature. The patient is ready to come off bypass when the haemodynamic condition is optimal. Clamp the venous line and remove the venous cannula. Oversew the tightened venous purse string site with a 4/0 polypropylene suture. Protamine sulphate is given to reverse the heparinization of the patient. The cardiotomy suckers from the pump oxygenator are removed.

Clamp the arterial line and remove the anchoring silk sutures. Remove the snugger of the aortic purse string and get ready to tie down the stitch when the assistant removes the aortic cannula. Check the suture line for bleeding and oversew with a 4/0 polypropylene suture.

After meticulous haemostasis of the operative field, place two drains. Bring out the anterior mediastinal and the pericardial (between the diaphragmatic pericardium and the inferior surface of the heart) drains through two separate stab wounds in the anterior chest wall below the xiphoid. When the mediastinum is dry, the chest is ready to be closed. Sometimes you may be able to approximate the pericardium loosely with interrupted sutures. Connect the drains to an underwater seal system. Ensure that the swab and instrument counts are correct before chest closure.

Place a large pack under the sternotomy. Approximate the two edges with stainless steel sternal wires (No. 5) mounted on a wire holder with Kocher's artery forceps on the other end of the wire. Pass four simple wire sutures round or through the body of the sternum and two through the manubrium. Remove the pack and twist the wires to bring the two edges together firmly. Turn the ends of the wires so that they are buried in the periosteum.

Approximate soft tissues, including the muscle and the linea alba, with continuous No. 2 PDS suture, followed by subcutaneous running suture and finally subcuticular 3/0 Vicryl stitch to close the skin.

Emergency reopening of sternum for severe bleeding and/or tamponade

Sudden massive haemorrhage or cardiac tamponade are life-threatening complications that require immediate reoperation in the

ITU. It is important to proceed immediately but also to call for senior help immediately. Blood loss must be replaced and more blood should be ordered.

Sudden increase in chest drainage and tamponade usually occurs within the first 12 hours postoperatively. Surgical instruments required are found in the cardiac bypass set on the intensive care unit. Good lighting is essential. Wire cutter, wire holders, extra Yankauer suckers, suction tubing and internal defibrillator must be available. This will get you started for the chest opening.

Procedure

Prepare and drape the skin with aqueous povidone-iodine solution. Place a green skin pack as close to the sternotomy as possible and hold it with towel clips. The rest of the draping is as for routine sternotomy unless indicated otherwise.

Remove the closing sutures with a skin knife and scissors. Lift up the ends of the sternal wires with curved artery forceps and cut them with a wire cutter. Place sternal retractors and release tamponade with suckers to remove blood clots. Have some 4/0 and 5/0 polypropylene sutures ready for any bleeder and systematically explore for any bleeding points. Check clotting times and correct any coagulopathy. Fresh frozen plasma and platelet infusions are usually required.

Once haemostasis is achieved with no evidence of further bleeding, place new chest drains if needed. Otherwise remove blood clots from the pre-existing chest drains by flushing with syringes of saline. Connect up the chest drainage system and close the sternotomy.

Harvesting the long saphenous vein for aortocoronary bypass grafts

Dissection of the long saphenous vein is one of the most important parts of the coronary bypass surgery. Atraumatic technique is essential to prevent intimal damage.

Procedure

Prepare both legs circumferentially from the medial malleolus to the thigh, and place them in a frog-like position with a soft flat pillow beneath the thighs. Wrap both feet in sterile towels, and apply steridrapes to both legs.

Identify the long saphenous vein 1 cm in front of the medial malleolus. Make a skin incision directly over the vein with a scalpel.

Use sharp scissors dissection to free the vein from the perivenous tissue.

Extend the incision upwards with the aid of finger dissection in the correct tissue plane next to the vein. Avoid excessive traction and direct grasping of the vein.

Tie and divide all branches between fine ligatures (3/0 braided silk) 1 mm away from the vein graft. If you are unsure of the presence of small venous side branches, divide the tissues well away from the vein to leave enough of the branch to be tied later. Sometimes it may be convenient to clip the distal end with a ligaclip. In the lower part of the leg, the long saphenous vein is in close proximity to the saphenous nerve. Try to identify and preserve the nerve.

Check the approximate length of the vein required for grafting. When the vein is totally mobilized, divide the distal (ankle) end of the harvested vein graft and cannulate it to ensure reversal of the saphenous vein. Gently dilate the vein with heparinized blood or Hartmann's solution. Excessive distension will cause intimal disruption. Ligate or suture any untied branches. Tie off the two *in situ* ends of the saphenous vein.

Meticulous haemostasis and avoidance of raising skin flaps while dissecting are essential for good healing of the donor leg wound. Close the leg before cardiopulmonary bypass with a Redivac drain (10 French) if indicated. Use subcutaneous absorbable 2/0 Dexon suture and subcuticular 3/0 Vicryl suture.

> Gently push the tips of the scissors into the tissue next to the vein and open them in the line of the vein to clear the perivenous tissue. Slide the scissors under the vein to clear behind it.

Preparation of the left internal mammary artery

The use of the left internal mammary artery (LIMA) to the left anterior descending coronary artery is associated with superior patency rates and longer survival when compared with saphenous vein graft. The right internal mammary artery can also be used for the appropriate coronary lesions.

Procedure

After median sternotomy, retract upwards the left chest wall using an adapted IMA retractor. Raise the operating table and rotate it away from you to facilitate dissection. Loupe magnification and good lighting help to visualize the small branches of the LIMA.

Harvest the LIMA as a pedicled graft from the first rib superiorly to beyond the LIMA bifurcation inferiorly. Strip away the left pleura and make a longitudinal incision in the endothoracic fascia 1 cm medial to the LIMA and veins. Commencing at the midpoint of the incision, gently free the LIMA, accompanying veins and perivascular tissue from the undersurface of rib cage using the tip of an unactivated cautery blade. Carefully dissect out intercostal branches, clip or cauterize them with coagulating current and divide them. From the first intercostal space upwards, do not use cautery to free the LIMA to avoid injury to the phrenic nerve.

After heparinization, divide and ligate the distal end of the LIMA. Assess its free flow. To minimize spasm, spray dilute papaverine solution (60 mg in 15 ml of Hartmann's solution) on to the LIMA graft throughout its whole length with a small syringe and size 25 needle. Control bleeding from any side branches with clips. Wrap the LIMA pedicle in a papaverine-soaked gauze and set it aside for use later. Finally, remove the IMA retractor.

Paediatric surgery

11

Mervyn Griffiths

HANDLING CHILDREN AND THEIR PARENTS

As a surgical SHO, you are unlikely to have your own children. You will therefore find it very difficult to appreciate the enormous stress felt by otherwise rational parents when their child is ill or needs an operation, however minor. It is not until your own child is ill that you can really empathize with parents. Every parent of a child in hospital is, by definition, anxious and worried and this anxiety may present in several different ways; the parents may be aggressive, dazed or tearful (especially immediately post-partum) and will almost certainly not take in all you say first time.

The surgical SHO has to be able to communicate, not only with the child but also with the parents. You will need to explain patiently, in language they can understand, and in a caring manner, what is needed and why, possibly on several occasions.

Neither the children, nor the parents are as easy to manage or bluff as an adult patient; the child will not let you hurt him/her more than once and the parents will fight much harder on behalf of their child than they would fight for themselves.

Outpatients

No small child can wait in an adult outpatient department for long without getting bored and troublesome. By the time they reach you they will be miserable and unexaminable. Ideally, therefore, you should persuade your consultant to see children in a dedicated clinic, which has suitable toys, books and diversions and which will convince the child that coming to hospital is 'a good thing'. If the child is dragged screaming from the clinic against his/her will, you have won.

Inpatient stay

This should be as short as possible, since most children come with their own potential nurse (the mother). Most minor paediatric surgical conditions can be treated as day cases, e.g. circumcision, herniotomy, orchidopexy, hydrocele, branchial anomalies and investigations such as sigmoidoscopy, cystoscopy, gastroscopy. A general anaesthetic is now so safe in the hands of an experienced anaesthetist that no child should be subjected to any invasive procedure under local anaesthetic if at all possible. The fear in the eyes of a 7-year-old who had the last chest drain put in under local anaesthetic when a second drain is suggested is not easily forgotten.

Children should be encouraged to visit the unit preoperatively if possible in order to reduce the stress of the actual admission. They need to bring a favourite toy or two, especially a 'Linus blanket'. Parents have to have adequate facilities to stay if they want to – an armchair is not good enough.

Postoperatively, adult patients have to be told what to do. In contrast, toddlers will not get out of bed if they do not want to, but will not stay in bed, except under duress, once they are well enough to get up.

Once children are eating, can walk to the toilet and their pulse and temperature are normal, they can be discharged home. Thus the average postoperative stay for children with appendicitis is less than 48 hours.

Never lie about postoperative pain to anyone, especially a child. If you do, the child will never trust you (nor many other adults) again. Explain that the wound is bound to hurt, but there are plenty of medicines (like Calpol) that will make the pain better.

No child over the age of 12 months should have any venepuncture, either for tests or an i.v. cannula, without first applying local anaesthetic cream at least 45 min previously. Only collapsed children are too ill to notice the pain. Similarly, intramuscular injections, unless through an indwelling i.m. cannula, are inhumane and should be avoided if at all possible. If the child cannot take medicines orally, most can be given rectally or intravenously by bolus or infusion.

History-taking

It is critical when taking a history from children to get their confidence, pitch your questions in terms they can understand ('poo', not 'bowel action') and don't let the parent answer on behalf of the child all the time. Above the age of 4, children can usually give an excellent description of the problem and will often have their own views on causation. Adolescents expect to be talked to as adults and should be. This may well require the parent to be restrained from replying, by means of a statement to the child such as, 'I'll talk to you about your pain first and then I will see if your mother wants to add anything'.

Grandparents often come to hospital as moral support, especially for single mothers. They should be allowed their say, but only after the child and the parent(s) have had theirs. This may require firmness.

Examination

Babies are best examined on a changing mat and the parents will be very impressed by a competent nappy replacer. A paediatrician is defined by some as a doctor who takes a nappy off and does not put it back on again. Babies need to be re-dressed promptly and not left exposed for ages as they can get cold easily.

Toddlers may be examined best on their mother's knee as an examination couch may be too frightening.

Older children with abdominal pain are acutely aware that examination will hurt. To gain their confidence small children should have their abdomen examined with their own hand first and subsequently by the doctor's hand. An attempt to demonstrate rebound tenderness is an assault and should never be attempted. Percussion of the abdomen is just as useful and not so painful.

Rectal examination is a potential minefield for SHOs. The adult aphorism 'you must always put your finger up or you will put your foot in it' relates to rectal carcinoma and is inappropriate for children. It is crucial not to have a blanket rule but to decide if the rectal examination is really necessary. In an ill child with 'barn door' appendicitis and guarding in the right iliac fossa, a rectal examination adds nothing to the decision to take the appendix out, which has already been made. However, if a child is ill, pyrexial, with a tachycardia but insufficient abdominal tenderness to explain the signs, then the rectal examination is mandatory to diagnose a pelvic appendix. Similarly, a rectum full of hard faeces can be diagnosed and treated with a bisacodyl suppository at the same examination.

Premedication

Most day cases do not require premedication if they have been adequately prepared for surgery. Many anaesthetists like to give children up to 1 year of age a premed of atropine ($20\mu g/kg$) intramuscularly 30 min preoperatively to prevent bradycardia on induction. Opiate premeds cause vomiting postoperatively.

Local anaesthetic

Practically all patients benefit from a 0.25% bupivacaine block. This can either be a regional block put in by the anaesthetist after induction, e.g. caudal epidural, ilioinguinal or ring block, or as a field block put in by the surgeon as the wound is closed.

> Ask your scrub nurse to remind you to put in the field block, as you will be keen to finish and write the operation note.

Temperature and blood loss

Small children and babies lose heat rapidly, so make sure that they are on a warming blanket in a warm theatre and their temperature is being monitored.

A 3 kg baby has a blood volume of 270 ml, so losing 25 ml of blood is significant. Blood loss needs to be monitored carefully and consciously kept to a minimum.

Crossmatch

Only the major operations require crossmatched blood. Because they are fewer, the blood is more easily forgotten. Ask the registrar or consultant every time you make up the operating list.

Blood tests

There is no such thing as a 'routine' blood test in children. Taking bloods from children – especially toddlers – is a major undertaking for phlebotomists, doctors and children alike.

Bloods should only be done if they are actually going to change management. For example, a white cell count is unlikely to influence the decision about an appendicectomy.

INTRAVENOUS FLUIDS AND INTRAVENOUS CANNULAS

Intravenous fluids

If in any doubt about the intravenous fluids required by a child, do not hesitate to ask the paediatric medical team, who are used to paediatric volumes. Do not, however, let them resuscitate a baby with pyloric stenosis using 0.18% saline with 4% dextrose as the baby will become severely hypokalaemic (see p. 249).

Maintenance fluids

Type: The standard maintenance fluid for children is 0.18% saline in 4% dextrose, with 1 g of KCl per 500 ml bag.

Postoperatively, the body conserves potassium actively and so for the first 24 hours do not include potassium in the maintenance fluid.

Volume: All paediatric volumes and dosages are related to body weight:

- 1–10 kg – 100 ml/kg/d, 4 ml/kg/h;
- the next 5 kg – 50 ml/kg/d, 2 ml/kg/h;
- thereafter – 20 ml/kg/d up to a maximum of 1500 ml/d in total.

For example:

- 10 kg – 1000 ml/d = 40 ml/h;
- 15 kg – 1250 ml/d = 50 ml/h;
- 32 kg – 1490 ml/d = 60 ml/h.

Dehydrated children may need more, but they are exceptional and should be managed in consultation with the paediatric team.

Replacement

All fluid losses, e.g. nasogastric aspirate, vomit, or losses into drainage bags, should be replaced millilitre for millilitre with 0.9% saline with 1 g KCl per 500 ml.

Postoperative hypovolaemia

This is easily measured non-invasively in children using the toe/core temperature difference, which should be less than 3°C. A wider difference should be treated with 4.5% HAS in 10 ml/kg boluses run in over 1–2 hours, repeated as necessary.

Intravenous cannulas

Accept that putting a drip up on a child will take longer than in adults and create the time to do it.

The most important item of equipment is an experienced paediatric nurse. She can look after the child, squeeze and restrain the limb, help fix the cannula and show you how to tidy up afterwards.

Surgical SHOs should not put up occasional drips on babies or allow themselves more than two attempts on a child – ask a skilled paediatric SHO to help you.

Local anaesthetic cream must be applied to several preinspected likely sites at least 45 min prior to the cannula insertion. This provides excellent anaesthesia, but a 3-year-old will still scream when s/he sees the needle.

If possible, take the child to a treatment room. This separates the child from the safe haven of his/her bed and from his/her parents, who will not be able to inhibit you by their presence. It also means that the screams are not heard by the other children on the ward.

> Practise putting cannulas into anaesthetized children who require a second or replacement cannula for i.v. access peroperatively.

> If no nurse is available, try again later.

Assemble all your equipment first: paper towel, sterets, cannulae, 'T-piece' preflushed with normal saline in a 2 ml syringe, splint and plenty of tape that sticks, e.g. pink zinc oxide tape, Transpore, Steri-Strips or Opsite, and blood specimen bottles if necessary.

Usually you can find a suitable vein on the back of the non-dominant or non-thumb-sucking hand or forearm. Only use the antecubital fossa if desperate – try the foot first, unless the child is mobile.

With the child's arm suitably secured by the paediatric nurse, place the paper towel under the arm to catch any mess. Wipe off the anaesthetic cream and clean the skin with an isopropyl alcohol swab. Holding the child's fingers with one hand, insert the cannula at 20° to the skin, aiming at a venous Y-junction . Flashback means that the tip of the needle, not the cannula, is in the vein so advance the needle at least 2 mm further (if you advance the cannula over the needle, this may push the vein off the needle – Fig. 11.1).

Then advance the cannula over the needle into the vein and withdraw the needle. Take the blood specimens prior to attaching the T-piece, then flush with normal saline. Secure the cannula without creating a tourniquet using both a chevron under the cannula, which is crossed proximally, and several pieces over the hub and T-piece. Try to fix it so that the insertion site is clearly visible to check for subsequent tissuing, though this may be impossible. The fixation of the tubing is critically important so that, when the child pulls on it, the force is taken by the tape well away from the cannula itself. Apply a crepe bandage and a plastic splint, which helps protect the cannula and prevents the child from using the limb normally. All this strapping decreases the likelihood that you both have to endure a repeat performance.

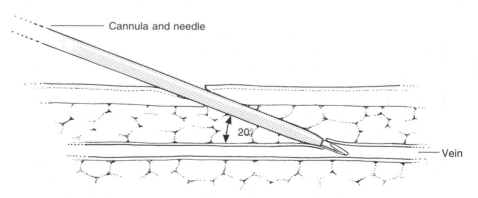

Fig. 11.1   Only the needle is in the vein, not the cannula.

Take the child back to his/her bed and parents and reward him/her with a suitable 'I've been brave' sticker.

PAEDIATRIC CIRCUMCISION

Definition

Circumcision is the excision of the foreskin, i.e. both the inner 'pseudomucosa' and the outer skin.

Natural history of the foreskin

At birth the foreskin (prepuce) is stuck to the glans by 'preputial adhesions' that protect the glans while the baby is incontinent. Between the ages of 3 and 14, the adhesions lyse and the foreskin becomes increasingly retractile. No postpubertal boy has adhesions, so they do not require any treatment. As the adhesions are lysing, bacteria can get underneath and infect the smegma produced by the glands around the glans. This causes balanitis and is sufficiently frequent to be normal. White, subpreputial collections of smegma (preputial pearls) are normal and will discharge when the adhesions lyse.

Before 3 years of age, it is impossible to assess whether the foreskin is non-retractile because of normal adhesions or because of a phimosis – a fibrous ring at the end of the foreskin preventing retraction. If a phimosis is present and all the adhesions have lysed, then the foreskin will balloon on micturition.

Indications

Circumcision is required for boys who cannot retract the foreskin to wash behind it. The operation effectively avoids any risk of sexual problems and penile carcinoma in adulthood.

The only universally agreed indication is balanitis xerotica obliterans (BXO), which causes a white, tight phimosis with underlying meatal stenosis in 6–12-year-olds, most of whom had previously had retractile foreskins.

A **phimosis** may be congenital (but undiagnosable until at least 3 years of age) or acquired as a result of recurrent balanitis.

Chronic recurrent balanitis causes scarring, radial lines of tiny white follicles on the foreskin and splitting on attempted retraction.

A **paraphimosis** is due to a phimosis that is large enough to allow the foreskin to be retracted, but too tight to permit replacement over the corona. A tourniquet-like effect results.

Social circumcision is practised in parts of the United States of America (up to 90% in some areas) and Australia (50% and dropping). Religious circumcision is compulsory for Jews and Muslims. Most primitive societies have a circumcision ritual. Trauma (caught in zip) leads to circumcision in a small group of boys who usually present with the trousers already cut off. The overall European circumcision rate is about 7%. In Denmark it is 1%.

Technique

Circumcision can always be done as a day case under general anaesthetic with a caudal or penile regional bupivacaine block.

Dilate the phimosis and retract the foreskin over the glans. Ensure that all the preputial adhesions have been freed up, especially ventrally on the corona. Replace the foreskin and apply two mosquito forceps, one dorsally and the other ventrally in the midline at the position of the tight ring. Pull the foreskin up at 45° and apply bone-cutters firmly and horizontally so that they just go over the tip of the glans, which you protect with your left thumb (Fig. 11.2).

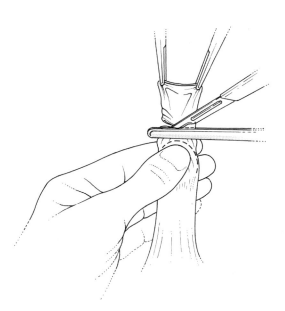

Fig. 11.2 The left thumb controls the position of the bone-cutters.

This ensures that the tight band is excised, but the shaft is not denuded. Cut off the excess foreskin using a number 10 blade.

Remove the bone-cutters, free the shaft skin from the pseudomucosa and push the skin proximally. Apply two mosquito forceps to the pseudomucosa dorsally and ventrally in the midline. Cut off the excess pseudomucosa with curved scissors, leaving 2–3 mm around the corona as a 'skirt'.

Ensure complete haemostasis with bipolar diathermy. Do not use unipolar diathermy. Suture the skin to the pseudomucosa with interrupted 5/0 catgut sutures starting with a dorsal stay suture. The ventral frenular stay stitch is U-shaped in order to transfix the frenulum and prevent bleeding from the frenular artery.

Cover the suture line with chloramphenicol eye ointment ('willy cream') to prevent sepsis and to stop the suture line sticking to anything.

> Hold the bone-cutters in your dominant hand and the scalpel in the other hand.

Postoperative care

Adequate analgesia with paracetamol elixir or diclofenac is a very variable requirement. Some boys prefer fresh air below the waist, while others prefer 'Y-front-type' pants to prevent movement. A period of 10 days off school is normal and is best managed by the Paediatric Community District Nurse.

Although most boys like to avoid baths for a week, a quick splash may be necessary if the suture line is very messy. A hairdryer on a low heat can be used in lieu of a towel.

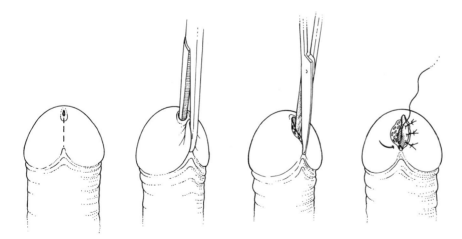

Fig. 11.3 Meatotomy.

Complications

Bleeding, infection and meatal stenosis are the commonest complications and may occur in 1–2% of cases. Immediate postoperative oozing may stop. If unchanged after a couple of hours, return the child to theatre and formally find the bleeding point – usually the frenular artery. Degloving is possible.

Balanitis xerotica obliterans has a 50% complication rate – mostly meatal stenosis. This can be 'avoided' by performing a pre-emptive meatotomy at the original operation. The meatus is crushed ventrally for 3–4 mm with straight mosquito forceps and then enlarged with scissors. The cut edges are sutured with one or two catgut sutures (5/0) each side to appose the urethral and glans epithelia (Fig. 11.3).

HERNIOTOMY

Definition

Herniotomy is the division (-tomy) of the hernial sac – without repair of the anterior abdominal wall (-rraphy).

Embryology

When the testis descends, a tube of peritoneum is dragged into the scrotum (or beside the round ligament into the labium majus). This processus vaginalis ensheaths the testis (*vagina* = 'scabbard') and is patent at birth in 50% of male full-term babies. Normally it obliterates, but if it stays open a little, then peritoneal fluid tracks down, collects around the testis and forms a hydrocele. If it is wide open then bowel can enter it (i.e. a hernia), and the processus vaginalis is called the 'hernial sac'.

Thus both hydrocele and hernia in children are due to failure of obliteration of the processus vaginalis, a congenital abnormality, and require the same operation – 'ligation of patent processus vaginalis' or 'herniotomy'. By definition all paediatric inguinal hernias are 'indirect'.

Indications

Hydroceles need ligation of the patent processus vaginalis (PPV) after 12 months as they will not obliterate after this.

Because of the risk of incarceration in paediatric hernias, all hernias need herniotomy, not conservative treatment. Babies less than 6 months old need repair within 2 weeks and older children within 8 weeks.

Operation

At least 90% of herniotomies can be performed as day cases.

Under general anaesthetic and an ilioinguinal bupivacaine block, make a 2 cm incision horizontally in the skin crease above the inguinal ligament medially from the femoral artery. Divide the fat, Scarpa's fascia and deeper loose connective tissue down to the external oblique aponeurosis (EOA).

Clean the EOA to ensure that you know exactly where you are. Dissect towards the scrotal neck to identify the shiny cord.

Incise the EOA in the line of its fibres and apply a mosquito forceps to each edge. Split the fibres proximally and distally to open the superficial inguinal ring (SIR; Fig. 11.4(**a**)).

Pick up the cord and strip the cremaster off so that all that remains is the processus, the vas and the vessels. Place a clip on the processus and stretch the cord over your finger. Using non-toothed forceps, strip the fascial layers off the processus taking the vas and vessels

> The EOA is the layer that does not move if you try to slide it about.

> Pull on the testis to see the cord move.

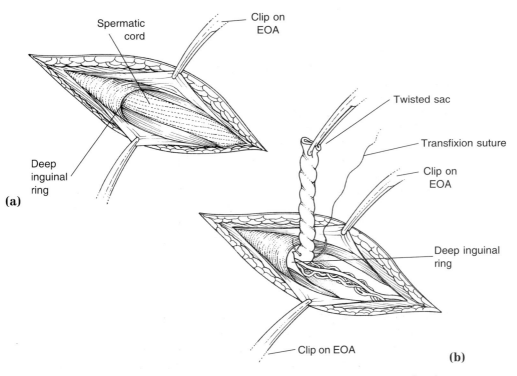

Fig. 11.4 (**a**) External oblique opened. (**b**) Sac divided and transfixed at deep inguinal ring.

> To reduce the risk of opening the processus, strip the fascia with a movement away from the cord.

with them. Keep going until all the fascia is freed and you reach your glove.

The processus may be diaphanous and dissecting off the vas and vessels may be extremely difficult even for an experienced paediatric surgeon. Do not be afraid to call for help if it begins to disintegrate.

Double-check that the vas and vessels are safe, then divide the processus between clips with scissors or diathermy. Retract the distal end (i.e. the testicular end) towards the midline to provide some tension and dissect the vas and vessels from the proximal end up to the deep inguinal ring. Twist the clip to ensure the sac is empty and transfix and ligate it with an absorbable suture (e.g. 4/0 Vicryl; Fig. 11.4(**b**)). First divide the suture and then divide the excess processus to ensure that the suture does not cut out. If it does, the sac will retract and you will have enormous problems retrieving it.

Check the distal end of the sac for bleeding and ensure that the testis is in the scrotum. Close the OEA with continuous absorbable sutures (e.g. 4/0 Vicryl) and then put two or three interrupted sutures in Scarpa's fascia. Close the skin with subcuticular 5/0 undyed Vicryl, Steri-Strips and Opsite. Check again that the testis is in the scrotum.

Complications

Recurrence is rare and is usually due to the transfixion suture coming off. Iatrogenic undescended testis can be avoided by checking that the testis is in the scrotum after you have closed the skin.

ORCHIDOPEXY

Definition

Orchidopexy is the fixation (-pexy) of the testis (orchido-) in the scrotum, usually following mobilization from an undescended position, but, pedantically, should also include simple 'fixation of testis' for torsion.

Natural history and indications

The testis is bilaterally descended in 97% of term boys and any undescended testes that are going to descend will do so by 6 months. However, at present, the recommendation is for an operation at 18 months as it is technically easier for the surgeon (and hence safer for the boy) and there are no visible histological changes on electron microscopy of the testis before then.

The problem in diagnosis is to separate normal, 'retractile' testes from real undescended testes. The former can be coaxed with ease to, at least, the midscrotum and will stay there when released. However, stroking the inner thigh causes cremasteric contraction and the testis pops back into the groin. Undescended testes have never been descended and cannot be manipulated into the scrotum at all, or only with enormous effort. There are twice as many orchidopexies performed as there are undescended testes, which implies that some 'retractile' testes are operated on in error. A very few testes are genuinely 'ascending', i.e. were descended at 6 months and then ascend as the processus vaginalis is reabsorbed into the anterior abdominal wall.

If a testis is impalpable and hence potentially intra-abdominal, it is important to retrieve it in order to ensure that, should it become malignant, this is diagnosed before it becomes the size of a grapefruit. If both testes are undescended then they must be operated on as spermatogenesis will be impaired, since the testes will be too hot in the groin. If, however, one testis is already descended and the other is readily palpable, then the only real indication for operation is cosmesis.

Operation

Most orchidopexies can be performed as day cases. Bilateral orchidopexies in boys over 10, groin exploration following laparoscopy and second-stage orchidopexy require admission overnight postoperatively.

Under general anaesthetic and an ilioinguinal bupivacaine block, expose the groin as for herniotomy. Using scissors, split the OEA in the line of its fibres to expose the entire inguinal canal from deep to superficial inguinal rings (Fig. 11.4). Pick up the testis and divide the gubernaculum with diathermy. Hold the testis up and strip off the cremasteric fibres to the deep inguinal ring. The cremasteric artery will need formal diathermy or it will ooze. Place a mosquito forceps on the tip of the testis or on the tip of the processus and give it to your assistant. Place a mosquito forceps on the processus itself and dissect it off the cord just as in a herniotomy (see above). Double check that the vas and vessels are safe before dividing the processus between clips. Retracting the cord medially makes dissection of the processus from the cord easier. Retract the deep inguinal ring laterally to ensure that the processus is freed as far as possible and transfix it with an absorbable suture (e.g. 4/0 Vicryl). With the deep inguinal ring held open by the retractor, dissect the peritoneum from the cord with a pledgelet until the vas can be seen to have separated medially from the vessels laterally. Pull the cord medially to put the 'lateral bands of Denis Browne' on the stretch before dividing them (Fig.

Aim to position the testis in the upper scrotum. Do not make life difficult by expecting it to go to the bottom of the scrotum every time.

11.5). Open and evert the distal processus to inspect the testis and epididymis.

Having checked that there is adequate cord length, tunnel your index finger from the groin incision into the scrotum and stretch the scrotal skin.

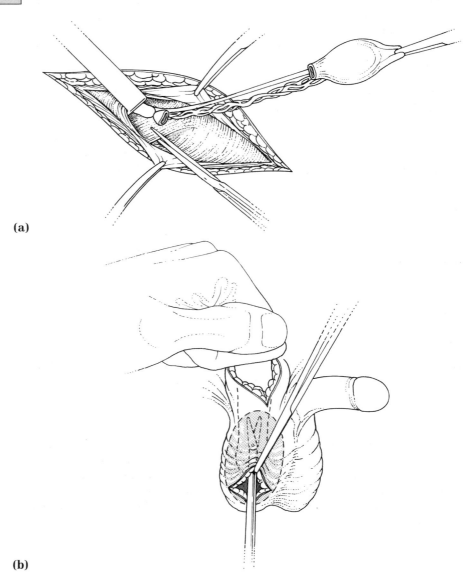

(a)

(b)

Fig. 11.5 **(a)** Scissors cutting the lateral bands of Denis Browne. **(b)** Creation of a dartos pouch. This technique is not appropriate in an adult.

Use the index finger of your left hand for a right orchidopexy and *vice versa*.

Incise just the skin of the scrotum. Make your assistant pick up one edge with toothed forceps and use iridectomy scissors to create a 'subdartos pouch'. Repeat for the other edge (Fig. 11.5).

Push a curved mosquito forceps through the scrotal incision and the scrotal fascia until its tip is on your scrotal index finger. Railroad the mosquito forceps into the groin as you withdraw your finger. Make sure that the cord and vessels are not twisted, grasp the testis and pull it down into the scrotal wound.

Place the testis and its coverings into the dartos pouch and close the skin with two 4/0 buried chromic catgut sutures, at least one of which should pick up the tunica albuginea of the testis.

Check the inguinal wound for bleeding and close it in layers, using an absorbable stitch (e.g. 4/0 Vicryl for the OEA and Scarpa's fascia and 5/0 undyed Vicryl for the subcuticular layer). Steri-Strips and Opsite hold the edges together and keep the wound clean.

Always make the pouch three times as big as you think you need, then placing the testis in it is easy.

Postoperative care

Check the wound and position of the testis at one month. An additional visit at 12 months is unnecessary in most cases or could be done by the child's general practitioner.

UMBILICAL HERNIA

Definition

The normal defect in the linea alba for the umbilical vessels is a potential hernia in everybody, but usually heals within 12 months.

Indications

Umbilical hernias never need repair unless they are more than 2 cm in diameter at 12 months of age or still present at 5 years. Children of sub-Saharan black African origin are especially prone to umbilical hernias, which are less likely to resolve spontaneously. Umbilical hernias virtually never cause problems in children, unlike inguinal hernias.

Operation

Make a 3 mm incision in the skin at the lower edge of the umbilicus. Insert the tip of a mosquito forceps and open it to split the skin

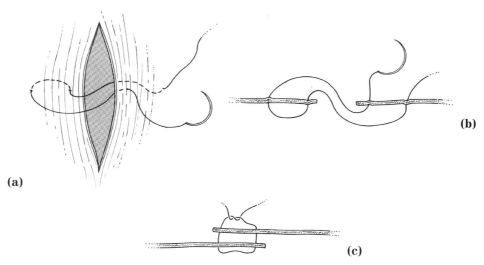

Fig. 11.6 Umbilical hernia repair. **(a)** Plan view. Three such sutures are usually enough. **(b)** Transverse section. The sutures are kept long until all have been placed. **(c)** Transverse section just before the knot is tied. The fascial layers overlap.

around the curve of the umbilicus. With mosquito forceps or curved scissors dissect around the sides of the hernial sac until it is freed circumferentially. Divide the sac from the skin and clear all the loose connective tissue from around the base to delineate the actual edges of the defect in the linea alba.

Use a double-breasted technique with two or three interrupted long-lasting sutures (e.g. 3/0 Maxon) or non-absorbable suture (e.g. 3/0 polypropylene) to minimize the chance of recurrence. Keep each untied suture long on a clip and tie them all at the end (Fig. 11.6).

The needle takes four bites of the wound edges. The sequence of the needle pass is not a simple in–out bite, but in–in–out–out:

- first bite: side A – far from the defect edge, outside–in (forehand stitch);
- second bite: side B – near to the defect edge, outside–in (backhand stitch);
- third bite: side B – far from the defect edge, inside–out (forehand stitch);
- fourth bite: side A – near to the defect edge, inside–out (backhand stitch).

Anchor the middle of the umbilical skin and close the wound with one interrupted 5/0 subcuticular undyed Vicryl suture.

Inject 0.25% bupivacaine around the umbilicus as a field block.

RAMSTEDT'S PYLOROMYOTOMY

Definition

Ramstedt's pyloromyotomy is the cutting or splitting (-tomy) of the muscle (-myo-) of the pylorus (pyloro-).

Indication

Infantile hypertrophic pyloric stenosis (IHPS) is probably the only condition to be treated by all surgeons throughout the world by the same operation – Ramstedt's pyloromyotomy.

Preoperative care

IHPS classically presents in a 10-day-old to 10-week-old baby boy who fed well at birth. Over 7–10 days the baby has increasingly frequent and vigorous vomits, culminating in full-blown 'projectile' vomits (across the room). (If the mother says her baby has 'projectile vomits' ask her what she does – she is probably a nurse.) The vomit is never bile-stained (i.e. not green), but may contain fresh or altered blood due to oesophagitis. The baby is usually hungry after the vomit and loses weight.

Metabolically, there is hyponatraemia, hypokalaemia, hypochloraemia and a metabolic alkalosis with dehydration. The baby needs to be resuscitated with 0.45% saline with 10% dextrose and 2 g KCl per 500 ml until the bicarbonate is less than 25 mmol/l and the chloride is greater than 90 mmol/l.

IHPS may be diagnosed by its two classical signs – the palpable pyloric tumour and visible peristalsis during a test feed. Ultrasonography is easier, and probably more accurate, if less shrouded with ritual.

After the biochemistry has been corrected, then is the time to operate – not before.

Empty the stomach with a nasogastric tube and leave it in place, replacing any aspirate millilitre for millilitre with 0.9% saline plus 1 g of KCl per 500 ml intravenously.

Anaesthesia

There is no place for local anaesthesia in the 1990s. Every hospital should have a designated anaesthetist and surgeon with a paediatric interest to whom these babies should be referred and if they are not present then the baby should be transferred to the nearest centre that has them.

Neonates lose heat rapidly, so the theatre needs to be warm (above 26°C), the baby needs to be on a warming blanket and the drapes and abdomen should be covered in Opsite to keep water out and heat in.

The operation

Use a 3–4 cm transverse muscle-cutting incision midway between the umbilicus and xiphoid right across the right rectus abdominis. Use diathermy to minimize the blood loss. Ligate and divide the umbilical vein. Identify the omentum, thence the transverse colon and thence the greater curve of the stomach. Deliver the fundus first and then work towards the antrum and pylorus, pushing down on either side of the wound to make the pylorus pop out. If the incision is too small, the delivery of the pylorus is traumatic or impossible. Using a gauze swab, make your assistant hold the antrum so that the relatively avascular area on the upper part of the pylorus is clearly displayed. Identify the actual length of the pylorus and incise the serosa only, starting 1–2 mm from the duodenal end. Continue across the pylorus and 1–1.5 cm on to the antrum (Fig. 11.7).

Reversing the scalpel, push the blunt end firmly into the wound over the proximal pylorus so that the muscle edges part. Then twist the scalpel through 90°, opening up the edges fully. Once the mucosa is bulging over the proximal pylorus, move on to the antrum and separate the edges proximally until the muscle appears to slide round at the apex of the incision. If necessary, incise a further 0.5 cm of serosa and separate some more. Finally, ensure that the pylorus is

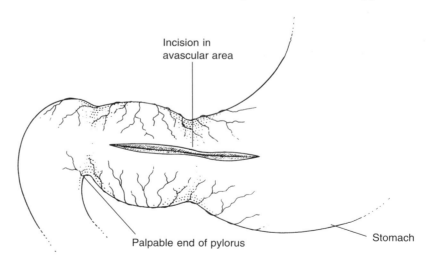

Fig. 11.7   The incision for pyloromyotomy. Note that it starts 2 mm from the palpable end of the pylorus and extends well up onto the antrum.

split distally, leaving 1 mm of palpable tumour unsplit. This will not effect the postoperative course, but will guarantee that the mucosa in the duodenal fornix is not breached.

Let a little blood collect in the muscular split and ask your anaesthetist to inflate 20–40 ml of air through the nasogastric tube. Force some through the pylorus into the duodenum and, if there is a leak, it will bubble through the blood.

To make a duodenal perforation is not a disaster, but to miss one may be. Any perforation should be oversewn with one 4/0 absorbable suture, buttressed with a piece of omentum. Close the wound in two layers with 3/0 or 4/0 absorbable continuous sutures using large non-ischaemic bites, remembering that this incision has a 1–5% dehiscence rate. Close the skin with absorbable subcuticular sutures, Steri-Strips and an Opsite dressing.

Inject 0.25% bupivacaine around the wound.

> An inadequate pyloromyotomy usually results from splitting the proximal two-thirds of the pylorus only with no splitting of the distal third or any extension on to the antrum.

Postoperative care

If there was no perforation, aspirate the air from the stomach and remove the nasogastric tube. Keep the baby on maintenance fluids overnight and start with full milk feeds at 9 am the next day. Special feeding regimens are unnecessary.

If there was a perforation, keep the nasogastric tube on free drainage and the baby nil by mouth for 48 hours, then feed a dextrose feed first, followed by full milk feeds if all is well.

Complications

Wound infection rates of 10–15% and dehiscence rates of 1–5% are common but unacceptable.

Urology

12

John Cumming

GENERAL PRINCIPLES IN SCROTAL SURGERY

Incision

To expose the testis, hold the testis between thumb and fingers stretching the scrotum over the testis. Make a 2–3 cm incision in the midline raphe and continue on to the testis until a small bead of clear fluid is seen. This shows that the tunica vaginalis has been incised. Extend the incision with scissors until the testis is delivered.

Haemostasis

Haemostasis is important to avoid haematoma formation. Diathermy of bleeding vessels in the cord is important but most postoperative bleeding appears to arise from the dartos layer.

Wound closure

The dartos muscle is the important layer to close as most postoperative haematomas occur from inadequate closure of this layer. The dartos muscle retracts under the wound margins and has to be picked up by the suture needle when closing this layer. Apply two Allis or similar tissue forceps to the dartos layer to bring it to the fore when closing the wound. Use absorbable sutures (polyglycholate preferably) on the tunica vaginalis, the dartos and subcuticular closure of the scrotal skin.

Postoperative anaesthesia/analgesia

A spermatic cord block will provide postoperative pain relief for up to 6 hours. Infiltrate 10 ml of 0.5% bupivacaine directly into the cord when the testis is exposed. Prescribe further analgesia with paracetamol or similar to start before the local anaesthetic has worn off. Subsequent doses may be taken as required.

Wound care

The scrotum has a good blood supply and healing is not usually a problem. Swelling and haematoma formation can be prevented by careful surgical technique. Suggest rest for the first 48 hours. The patient should be horizontal for most of this time and a scrotal support for a fortnight is advisable. The dressing may be soaked off in a bath on the morning after the operation. If catgut has been used in the skin/subcutaneous closure, a foreign body reaction is set up to absorb the material and the knot and suture often presents itself through the wound. Remove the suture to speed healing. (Some surgeons advocate interrupted skin closure with catgut, which is best removed after 5–7 days.)

HYDROCELES AND EPIDIDYMAL CYSTS

Indications

The presence of an epididymal cyst or a hydrocele is not an absolute indication for surgery. Aspiration affords short-term relief of the swelling. Surgery should be offered for symptomatic swellings. Request an ultrasound examination of the testis if there is any doubt of the testis itself.

Aims of surgery

Explain to the patient that excision of epididymal cysts does not prevent further cysts from developing. Also explain that an injury to the epididymis might result from excision of epididymal cysts and this would be equivalent to a vasectomy on the affected side. The implication to fertility might be important in younger men. Conversely, prevention of further epididymal cysts requires excision of the whole epididymis and this may be indicated in some men, especially with recurrent cysts.

Procedure

Hold the affected testis in the left hand and make a midline incision in the scrotum. Incise through dartos and the tunica. Expose the testis and examine the testis and epididymis. If there are any associated epididymal cysts, excise them if necessary. Incising the tunica of the hydrocele will immediately drain the hydrocele itself. Preventing a recurrence of the fluid is the object of the two procedures: **Lord's plication** is useful for the thick-walled and inflamed cyst. The tunica is plicated around the periphery so as to prevent the tunica from closing over the testis.

Use a continuous suture all along the free cut edge of tunica to reduce postoperative bleeding.

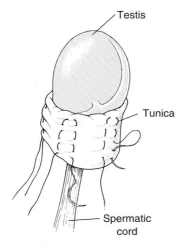

Fig. 12.1 Lord's plication for hydrocele.

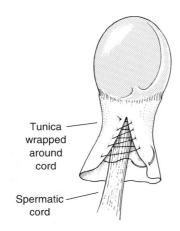

Fig. 12.2 Jaboulay's operation for hydrocele.

Evert the tunica around the testis and place four to six sutures to fold up the tunica in a rim behind the testis. Start at the edge of the tunica, pick up several bites of tissue and repeat the process from the testis to the edge of the tunica before tying the sutures (Fig. 12.1).

Jaboulay's operation is useful for the thin-walled tunica that will wrap comfortably around the spermatic cord under the testis. A few sutures will hold this in place (Fig. 12.2).

Make only a small incision in the tunica and evert the tunica fully. The tunica should roll up round the cord like a sleeve. Close the incision snugly around the cord.

CIRCUMCISION

Aims

Circumcision is the surgical removal of the foreskin. Apart from religious reasons, the commonest indication is phimosis. When circumcision is carried out for cancer of the foreskin a variation in the technique is required.

Anaesthesia

A general anaesthetic is usual but circumcision can be performed under local anaesthesia with or without sedation and a penile block is an effective adjunct to general anaesthesia for postoperative pain control. The dorsal nerves of the penis begin to fan out at the base of the penis and run superficial to the tough tunica of the corpora cavernosa. 0.5% bupivacaine provides anaesthesia for 4–6 hours postoperatively. If local anaesthesia is the sole anaesthetic agent then a second infiltration on the ventral surface around the corpus spongiosum is required to block the nerves travelling with the urethra. This latter infiltration is useful for frenuloplasty too.

The incision

Most mistakes over circumcision are made over placing the incision: usually insufficient skin is excised. Attach two artery forceps to the tip of the foreskin and stretch the foreskin. The corona of the glans is visible beneath the skin. Incise the shaft skin at this level (Fig. 12.3(a)).

Reposition the artery forceps on the distal margin of the incision and put it under tension. Separate the foreskin from the deeper tissues with a scalpel and blunt dissection with a swab. Remove only the skin (Fig. 12.3(b)). When your mobilization has reached the corona, excise the foreskin with scissors starting at the ventral surface of the everted skin tube and cutting down one side of the frenulum. Leave approximately 5 mm of inner foreskin cuff around the corona.

The frenulum

The frenulum frequently appears tight when the foreskin is retracted. Relieve this at the time of circumcision by dividing the frenulum close to the ventral surface of the glans penis. Leave it unsutured when the wound is closed (Fig. 12.3(c)).

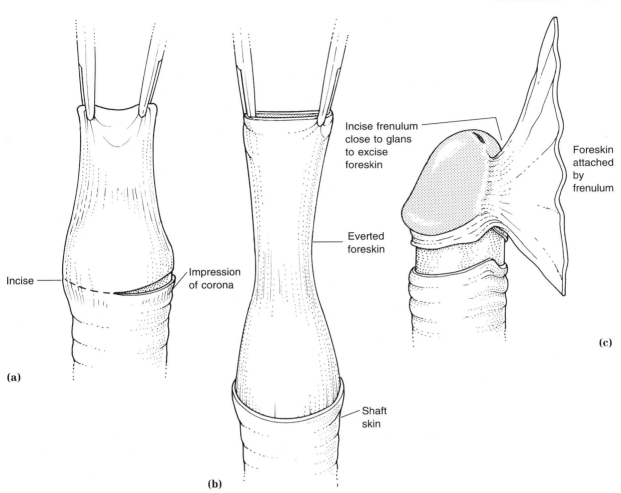

Fig. 12.3 Technique of circumcision. **(a)** Incise at level of corona. **(b)** Turn the foreskin inside out. **(c)** Incise the frenulum with scissors.

Circumcision for cancer of the foreskin

When a cancer is present it is important to remove the whole fore-skin, including the cancer and a margin of normal skin. Make the skin incision at the level of the corona before commencing the cir-cumcision. Apply two artery forceps to the end of the foreskin and open the foreskin with scissors, avoiding the cancer (Fig. 12.4). Excise the foreskin by continuing the incision around the penis, taking care to leave a 3–5 mm margin of healthy foreskin around the corona.

Haemostasis

Use bipolar diathermy for haemostasis on the penis. Subcutaneous veins may be transected but do not appear to be bleeding at the time of the operation. These should be cauterized or ligated with a 3/0 absorbable suture. In the technique of stripping the subcutaneous tissues from the foreskin described above most of the larger veins are avoided. Expose the frenular arteries and apply diathermy before cutting them.

Closure

A continuous subcuticular absorbable suture gives a satisfactory wound that heals rapidly. Take care not to draw the suture tightly as you close the wound or a tight ring scar can be produced. If interrupted absorbable sutures are used remove them after 5–7 days to avoid the foreign-body reaction mentioned above under 'General principles'.

> Do not use unipolar diathermy. This has particular hazards when applied to the penis. A diathermy burn of the whole penis can result when unipolar diathermy is used, especially in children.

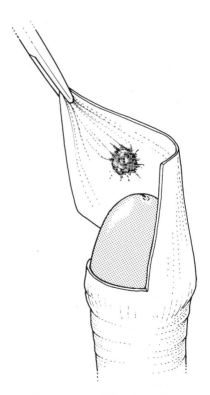

Fig. 12.4   Circumcision for cancer of the foreskin.

Aftercare

Apply a non-adherent dressing, which may be soaked off in a bath the day after the operation. Tell adult patients to avoid sexual intercourse for 6 weeks. Advise the patient to commence analgesia before the local anaesthetic wears off and continue regular doses for a few days. Ensure the patient has passed urine before he leaves the ward or day unit.

VARICOCELE

Indications

Operation for varicocele is indicated mainly for the symptoms of dragging and aching that occur with larger varicoceles. There is a controversial place for ligation of a varicocele in oligospermic subfertile men.

Aims of surgery

Ligation of the dilated spermatic veins should in theory result in thrombosis and obliteration of the veins. However, there may be numerous small anastomoses above and below the site of ligation, which gives rise to a significant recurrence rate. The veins can be exposed through a groin incision opening the inguinal canal. This has the advantage of being more familiar territory but there are many more veins and the testicular artery is more likely to be injured. Probably the better site to ligate the spermatic veins is just deep to the internal inguinal ring through a gridiron incision – the high ligation. Venous embolization under radiological screening is an alternative that should be considered.

Procedure (the high ligation)

Identify the internal ring at the midinguinal point half way between the symphysis pubis medially and the anterior superior iliac spine laterally. Place the incision 2–3 cm above and lateral to this point. Use a muscle-splitting 'gridiron' approach and enter the retroperitoneal space. Identify the dilated spermatic vein(s) as the cord passes through the internal ring and ligate and divide them. This approach has the benefit that the veins are larger and fewer in number.

> When the retroperitoneal space is entered, the spermatic veins tend to be attached to the peritoneum, which is retracted anteriorly. This can help you find the veins in the more obese patient.

Closure

Close the external oblique with absorbable suture and insert a subcuticular skin closure. No drain is necessary.

VASECTOMY

Indications

Vasectomy is an operation for male sterilization and as such should be considered to be irreversible. The patient should be warned that the reservoirs of sperm should be emptied and contraception should continue until there have been two consecutive negative semen analyses. There is a small risk of recanalization (1:2500) and rarely a third vas deferens may be missed and may account for persisting spermatozoa. Some men may complain of aching in the testes after vasectomy.

Aims of surgery

The operation consists of cutting and tying both vasa deferentia.

Procedure

Infiltrate 1 ml of 2% lignocaine into the scrotal skin in the midline anteriorly. Make a 1–2 cm incision through skin and dartos. Feel the vas with one finger behind the scrotum and your thumb in the wound, which makes it easier to find the vas (Fig. 12.5(a)).

Infiltrate further local anaesthetic around the vas and cord and place a tissue forceps around the vas and bring it to the surface. Incise the surface of the tissue overlying the vas until the surface of the vas glistens. Pass a fine artery forceps beneath the vas and mobilize the vas with blunt dissection. Place three artery forceps across the loop of vas and divide the vas between the proximal two forceps (Fig. 12.5(b)). Ligate the proximal end and doubly ligate the distal end using the two pairs of forceps (Fig. 12.5(c)). Further separate the two ends by burying the proximal cut end in the spermatic fascia.

> With gentle traction on the testis, start palpating for the vas in the midline and slowly sweep the finger and thumb laterally until the vas deferens is located.

> With the midline incision, be careful to identify both vasa separately and do not cut the same vas twice.

Wound care

Apply a gauze dressing to the scrotum and tell the patient to wear tight underpants for 24 hours. The dressing may be soaked off the following day in the bath. Scrotal support should continue for a fortnight.

Semen analysis

Contraception should continue until two consecutive negative sperm tests have been obtained. The first test is usually performed after 10–

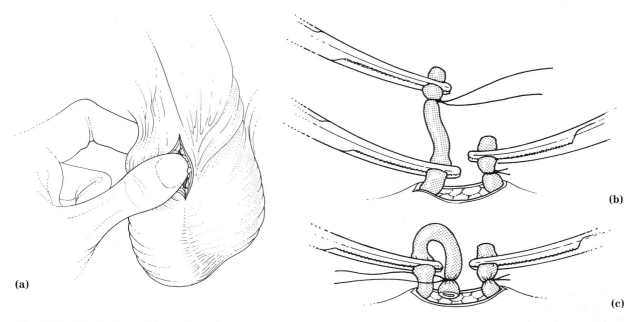

(a)

(b)

(c)

Fig. 12.5   Technique of vasectomy.

12 weeks. Tell the patient it usually takes 25 ejaculations to clear the system.

TESTICULAR BIOPSY

Indications

Testicular biopsy is indicated in the investigation of some infertility and contralateral testicular malignancy.

Procedure

Make a midline scrotal incision and, without changing your grip on the testis, make a 1 cm incision in the tunica of the testis to allow the seminiferous tubules to protrude. Excise the protruding seminiferous tubules with scissors and preserve the biopsy in Bouin's solution.

Haemostasis

Close the testis and then the tunica vaginalis with continuous absorbable sutures.

VASOGRAPHY

Indications

Vasography is indicated in obstructive azoospermia.

Procedure

Identify the spermatic cord and deliver the testis and cord through a midline scrotal incision. Take the opportunity to examine the epididymis. In obstruction, the dilated duct of the epididymis can be seen with the naked eye. Locate the vas, incise the adventitia over its surface and control the vas with an Allis forceps. Make sure the X-ray plate is situated properly and the radiographer is ready to expose the film. Insert a 25 gauge needle into the vas along its longitudinal axis aiming proximally (Fig. 12.6).

Gently apply pressure to the syringe plunger and, when the resistance drops, inject 1 ml of water-soluble radio-opaque solution. Observe carefully for distension or ballooning, which indicates extravasation. Expose the X-ray plate and repeat the procedure on the opposite side. The contrast should define the vas, outline the seminal vesicles and enter the prostatic urethra and bladder.

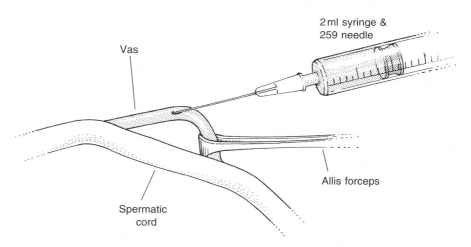

Fig. 12.6 Technique for vasography.

EXPLORATION AND REPAIR OF TRAUMA TO TESTIS

Indications

Substantial trauma to the testis results in bruising and swelling. The testis may be severely damaged or ruptured. Urgent ultrasonography will show the damage and a tunical tear may be worth repairing.

Aims of surgery

Surgical debridement and wound toilet may be required. Repair of the tunica albuginea is important to prevent sperm coming into contact with the body tissues and the (theoretical) risk of antibody development. Although the swelling may be large from haematoma and oedema there is often little blood clot to remove.

Incision

Use a midline scrotal incision and avoid traumatized scrotal skin if possible. Incise the tunica vaginalis and deliver the testis through the wound.

Procedure

Remove dead/damaged tissue, blood clot and foreign material. Examine the testis to assess viability and excise the testis if the blood supply is compromised. Repair the tunica of the testis with an absorbable suture, e.g. 3/0 polyglycolic acid.

Haemostasis

Haemostasis is important. Achieved this with diathermy or by underrunning a bleeding area with 3/0 polyglycolic acid suture. Drains to the scrotum are more likely to introduce more infection than to allow drainage of haematoma. Use one only for the drainage of purulent discharge (more likely when there has been considerable delay since injury took place, especially in the presence of ischaemic/necrotic tissue or a foreign body).

Wound closure

Close the dartos muscle layer with an absorbable suture such as polyglycolic acid or catgut. If you have any concern about contamination or infection leave the skin unsutured.

Postoperative analgesia

Local anaesthetic infiltration of the spermatic cord is an effective analgesic. Infiltrate away from the wound or injury. Palpate the spermatic cord at the neck of the scrotum between finger and thumb and immobilize it against the pubis. Infiltrate 5–10 ml of 0.5% bupivacaine into the cord. Paracetamol 1 g as required orally may be taken over the following days and an initial opiate analgesic is effective in the early postoperative period.

Wound care

A daily bath and change of dressing is the minimum necessary. More frequent dressings may be required for purulent discharge. Advise the patient to wear a scrotal support for a fortnight.

General surgery

13

Colin D. Johnson

This chapter will cover the general surgical procedures you might reasonably expect to perform as a trainee. You should read up the techniques of more complex procedures in a textbook of operative surgery (such as *Rob and Smith's Operative Surgery*) before you assist at them so that you understand the procedure and can follow the surgeon's line of action.

INCISION AND DRAINAGE OF ABSCESS

An abscess is a collection of pus within soft tissues. There will be surrounding erythema and oedema but unless the abscess is small there will be an obvious central softening.

Treatment of an abscess is incision and drainage of its contents. Surrounding cellulitis may require antibiotic treatment. Abscesses should be drained under general anaesthetic. Adequate analgesia is difficult to obtain with a local field block.

Operative technique

Clean and prepare the area of the abscess and ensure that all its possible extensions are accessible. Aspirate a sample of pus. Incise the skin over the softest, most fluctuant area of the abscess. If it has already pointed (obvious skin necrosis) or begun to discharge, use this area as the centre of your incision. Usually a single incision is sufficient and it is not necessary to make lateral extensions. For a superficial abscess it may be necessary to excise necrotic skin to 'saucerize' the abscess, whereas for a deep abscess with intact fascial layers over it a short incision is usually sufficient (Fig. 13.1).

Particularly for a deep abscess, ensure that all internal loculations are broken down. Insert two fingers through the incision and palpate all of the wall of the abscess cavity. Always send a sample of pus for culture. The microbiologist will prefer to have a sample of pus rather than swabs.

> To get a sample of pus uncontaminated by blood, aspirate the abscess using a white needle and a 10 ml syringe before making the incision. If this is not practical, obtain a sample of pus directly into the sterile container when you have incised the abscess. Make sure a bottle is available before you make the incision.

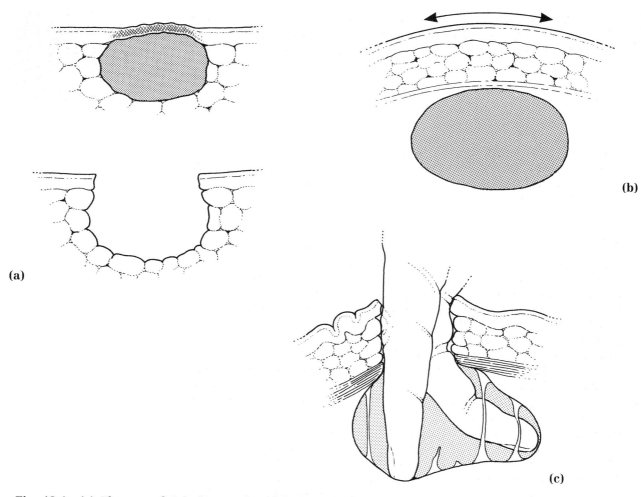

Fig. 13.1 **(a)** The superficial abscess should be 'saucerized' to open it widely. Excise any necrotic skin (shaded area) completely. **(b)** A deep abscess should be incised along its length (arrow). A single incision is usually sufficient. **(c)** Break down loculations by inserting two fingers into the cavity.

Haemostasis is not usually a problem. Control bleeding on the edge of the incision with diathermy. Blood vessels in the abscess wall will have thrombosed and rarely bleed.

After drainage, a superficial abscess should be loosely dressed with the widest ribbon gauze that will fit comfortably in the incision. Use only one or two folds to keep the skin edges apart and to serve as a capillary drain for exudate. Apply an absorbent dressing over the ribbon gauze.

Prescribe adequate postoperative analgesia. Change the dressing after 12–24 hours and then daily. At the first dressing change make sure that whole abscess has been drained and that surrounding cellulitis is receding.

Do not pack the abscess tightly. This prevents easy drainage, delays collapse of the cavity and is painful to remove.

Special sites

Axilla

Place the incision transversely across the axilla. There may be a deep communication, so explore the cavity with care. Place the patient's arm horizontally, at 90° to the trunk, to avoid tension on the axillary structures during operation.

Cervical

These abscesses are usually secondary to infected lymph nodes and occasionally to a brachial cyst. Do not attempt to operate on them unless you are confident of your knowledge of anatomical structures in this region, particularly the path of the relevant cranial nerves. Consider tuberculosis in the differential diagnosis and make sure you send separate specimens of pus and abscess wall for TB culture. Always obtain a specimen for histology.

Make a short incision over the abscess. Usually a curving skin crease incision is best in the neck, but sometimes a straight vertical or oblique incision will be more appropriate. Discuss this with a senior colleague. The incision should be relatively small. Deepen the incision through the fascia till you enter the abscess. For small abscesses, and where you are concerned for the safety of adjacent structures, make a stab incision on the most prominent part of the abscess. Insert a closed, blunt clip into the cavity and open it to increase the size of the incision. This will achieve drainage while protecting adjacent structures. Insert one finger or a blunt clip to ensure that loculations are broken down and insert a small corrugated drain. Use a Portex drain and cut a width of two or three corrugations appropriate to the size of the abscess. Attach the drain with a single suture to the skin and cover the wound with an absorbent dressing.

The inflammation usually settles rapidly and the drain can be removed after 2–3 days.

Breast

Most breast abscesses are related to lactation or puberty. They usually respond to antibiotic treatment. If this has failed, incise over

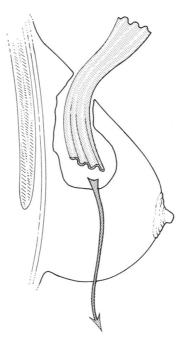

Fig. 13.2 A large, deeply placed breast abscess may (rarely) require a second incision to achieve adequate drainage.

the most obvious part of the abscess, using a radial incision lateral to the nipple and a transverse incision above and below the nipple. Insert one or two fingers and ensure all loculations are broken down. In a large breast, the abscess may be deep and surprisingly extensive.

Ensure that your incision has achieved adequate drainage of the cavity. If the cavity is extensive consider whether a second incision should be made to ensure dependent drainage (Fig. 13.2). This is rarely necessary. Place a corrugated drain into the cavity, and cover the wound with an absorbent dressing. Provide firm support with an appropriate brassiere and continue antibiotic treatment. The drainage should stop rapidly and you will be able to remove the drain after 48 hours.

Perianal abscess

Perianal abscesses can be divided into two groups, true perianal abscess and ischiorectal abscess (Fig. 13.3).

The treatment of the two groups is broadly similar. Incision and

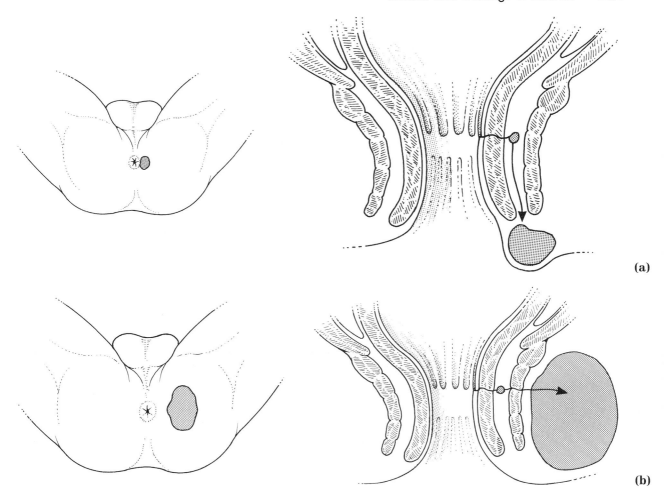

Fig. 13.3 **(a)** A perianal abscess presents at the anal margin. It results from infection in an anal gland tracking in the intersphincteric plane to reach the skin. **(b)** An ischiorectal abscess is more lateral and larger. It results from infection tracking from an infected gland laterally into the ischiorectal space. Both types of abscess require incision and complete drainage. The fistula is usually impossible to identify at acute presentation.

drainage should not be delayed because this may lead to necrotizing fasciitis. Place the patient in the lithotomy position under general anaesthesia. Incise over the most prominent area of the abscess and insert a finger into the cavity to break down loculations. These may be extensive in an ischiorectal abscess. Perianal abscesses are usually fairly superficial.

It is mandatory to collect a specimen of pus for culture. The presence of organisms of bowel origin indicates a high likelihood of fistula and the patient will require a subsequent examination under anaesthesia.

Do not attempt to identify any fistula track when draining an abscess. Oedema may obscure the internal opening and will make laying open the fistula more difficult. Content yourself with incision and drainage, but warn the patient before operation that a subsequent procedure may be necessary in 7–10 days to deal with any associated fistula.

Insert a ribbon gauze loosely into the cavity, bringing one or two folds out to serve as a capillary drain, and apply padding. Inspect the wound yourself 12–18 hours after operation and if there is evidence of progressive cellulitis make urgent arrangements for the patient to have another examination under anaesthetic by a senior colleague. Delay may result in extensive gangrene. Arrange for the dressing to be changed on the ward 12–24 hours after operation with adequate analgesia using opiates or nitrous oxide and oxygen. Subsequent dressing changes should be done daily at the patient's home or general practice surgery.

Remember to check the results of culture of the pus and arrange further examination under anaesthesia if necessary.

EXCISION OF MINOR LESIONS

Excision of skin lesions and sebaceous cysts is described in Chapter 9.

Lipoma

Position the patient comfortably with the lipoma in an accessible position. Use general anaesthesia for lipomas on the back of the neck or back of the trunk, where fibrous adhesions make excision difficult and where the thickness of the skin makes local anaesthesia difficult. In other sites, use local anaesthesia.

Infiltrate the skin over the lipoma and into the subcutaneous tissue around it. A large lipoma on the trunk will require an incision almost as long as the lesion. Deepen the incision through the dermis until you see the capsule of the lipoma. The fat often has an orangey tint. Elevate the skin edge with a skin hook and using sharp dissection with scissors divide the attachments between the lipoma and the dermis (Fig. 13.4).

Separate the skin from the underlying lipoma as far as the edge of the tumour. Then separate the other skin flap and continue the

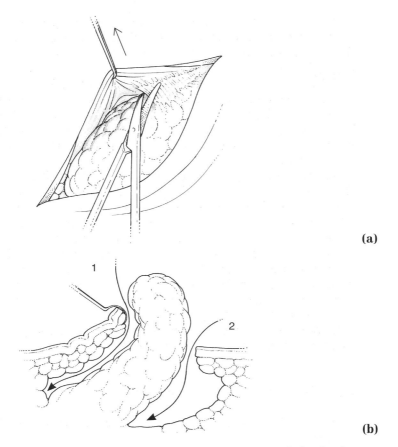

(a)

(b)

Fig. 13.4 Excision of lipoma. **(a)** Elevate one skin margin and divide the fibrous strands that attach the superficial aspect of the lipoma to the surrounding tissue. **(b)** When the lipoma has been cleared superficially all round (1), elevate one edge out of the wound and separate all of the deep attachments (2).

dissection round beneath the lipoma. Usually this will be an obvious plane and you will need to divide only a few fibrous strands as you go. Lift the lipoma up into the wound and complete the dissection on the deep surface (Fig. 13.4).

On the limbs, lipomas may be 'popped out'. Infiltrate over the lipoma and incise the skin (in the lines of skin tension, usually circumferential or oblique). The incision can be shorter than the tumour diameter. Separate the skin edges from the upper surface of the lipoma, then squeeze the lipoma on each side to force it up into the incision. Its peripheral attachments are often flimsy and it will pop out into the wound (Fig. 13.5).

> Handle the lipoma gently with a finger or a swab to avoid splitting its capsule. Look out for lobulated extensions into the surrounding tissue and ensure you remove these in continuity.

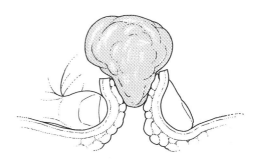

Fig. 13.5 'Popping out' a lipoma. After freeing the superficial surface, squeeze with finger and thumb to force the lipoma up and out through the incision. This technique is useful for small lipomas on the limbs.

Lymph node biopsy

Always carry out lymph node biopsy under general anaesthesia. It is a mistake to attempt this operation under local anaesthesia, however easily palpable the lymph node feels. It is always more difficult to find once you have cut the skin.

Site the incision over the lymph node, in a skin crease. In some sites such as the neck or the groin bear in mind possible subsequent incisions for block dissection (Chapter 7).

Incise through the skin and subcutaneous tissue down to the fascia. Secure haemostasis. Divide the fascia and separate it and the tissues beneath gently using a blunt forceps. Identify the abnormal node and lift up the deep fascia over it to facilitate dissection. Maintain traction on the surrounding tissues and incise gently around the lymph node with scissors.

Separate the attachments of the lymph node all round. Look for the hilar vessels and control these with diathermy. Lift the node up by its adventitia and complete the dissection of its deep surface.

Remember to take appropriate samples for bacteriology when required.

> Avoid grasping the lymph node with forceps, which destroys the architecture and makes histological evaluation more difficult.

> Consult the laboratory before you start, to find out if they wish the node sent fixed in formalin or fresh directly to the laboratory.

HIDRADENITIS SUPPURATIVA

The infected sweat glands in the axilla or groin can be excised under local anaesthetic. These often form a linear array of red inflamed tissue. Infiltrate around the inflamed area with local anaesthetic and excise the diseased skin on a narrow ellipse leaving the subcutaneous fact intact. Close the wound as described in Chapter 1.

Give the patient a broad-spectrum antibiotic with activity against staphylococci for five days. Close the wound with monofilament suture and remove the sutures after 10 days.

> Warn the patient that this is a frequently recurrent condition and further excisions are likely.

GANGLION

See Chapter 5.

INGROWING TOENAIL

Operations on ingrowing toenails are required when the nail bed becomes distorted and the nail grows into the edge of the nail fold. Cellulitis and suppuration result. If conservative measures such as elevation of the nail edge with a piece of cotton wool tucked under the nail have failed, surgical treatment will be necessary.

If there is severe infection and swelling it may be best to perform preliminary avulsion of the nail before definitive surgery. Complete the surgical treatment by lateral excision of the nail bed when the inflammation has settled.

Lateral excision of the nail bed

Most cases of ingrowing toenail can be dealt with by excision of the lateral portion of the nail and nail bed, without removing the whole nail. It is possible to deal with both edges of one nail although this may leave a narrow remnant. There is disagreement among surgeons over the relative merits of surgical excision of the nail bed or application of phenol. The lowest recurrence rates are achieved with a combination of both techniques.

Insert a digital ring block (Chapter 2). Use plain 1% lignocaine, for rapid onset of action without dangerous vasoconstriction. Apply a rubber tourniquet (use a 10 or 12 French Jaques catheter). Wrap the catheter twice around the base of the toe and secure it with a clip to occlude the blood supply.

> Do not tie the catheter. Secure it with a clip so that you do not forget to remove it at the end of the procedure.

With a pair of heavy, straight scissors cut down the nail close to the ingrowing edge, but on the flat part of the nail plate. Remove the lateral portion of nail with a heavy artery forceps (Fig. 13.6).

Take a small, round-bladed scalpel (No. 15) and incise the skin over the nail bed in the same line as the nail cut. Incise the skin laterally to skirt the margins of the nail fold (Fig. 13.6). Deepen the medial line of incision through the nail bed and try to remove the lateral margin of the nail bed and nail fold intact. If you accidentally cut across the deepest portion of the nail bed, grasp the remaining tissues in a pair of fine toothed forceps and excise it from the bone with the scalpel. Failure to do this will result in a recurrent spike of nail.

Next apply phenol. Use aqueous 5% phenol. Dip a cotton bud into the phenol and press it into the nail fold for 1 min. Wipe away any

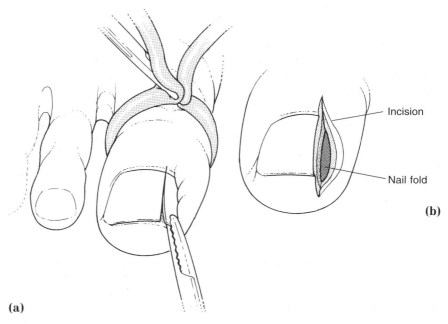

Fig. 13.6   Lateral excision of the nail bed for ingrowing toenail. **(a)** After cutting the affected edge of the nail, grasp the lateral portion with a heavy forceps and pull it up and away. **(b)** Extend the incision over the nail fold and laterally to excise all granulation tissue. Deepen this to include the full recess of the nail fold.

excess that gets on the skin to avoid a caustic burn. Remove the cotton bud and flood the area with ethyl alcohol to neutralize the phenol.

No sutures are required. Wrap a piece of paraffin gauze around the toe, leaving the end exposed, and then wrap a piece of dressing gauze around the toe. Take a three-ply gauze square. Unfold one layer to make a rectangle. Fold this in half lengthways and wrap it round the toe leaving the end exposed. Place the thicker half of the gauze over the operated side of the toe. The dressing will go round about one and a half times. Then hold the gauze in place with a few turns of 2 inch elasticized gauze. At this point you must remove the rubber tourniquet. If you have held it in place with a clip that will remind you to remove it. Continue the gauze roll up on to the forefoot and, after a couple of turns, back on to the toe before coming back on to the foot to secure the dressing.

Complete the operation by checking the colour of the end of the toe and confirm the presence of rapid capillary refill.

> The padding around the toe need not be very bulky, but it should be firm enough to control bleeding while not occluding the circulation.

APPENDICECTOMY

Appendicectomy is indicated for patients with right iliac fossa pain in whom a reasonable suspicion of acute appendicitis exists. The primary aim of the operation is to remove the appendix. For this a short incision is sufficient, but the diagnosis and treatment of other pathology may require considerable enlargement of the wound.

All women of childbearing age, and others in whom the diagnosis is in doubt, should undergo laparoscopy to make the diagnosis. If the appendix cannot be visualized, or if there is free fluid in the right iliac fossa or pelvis, perform appendicectomy. After laparoscopy it is possible to locate the incision accurately over the base of the appendix.

Operation

Make a 2–3 cm incision in the lines of skin tension, immediately below McBurney's point at the level of the anterior superior iliac spine. Alternatively, select the most appropriate site by laparoscopy. Incise the subcutaneous fat and clean the external oblique aponeurosis.

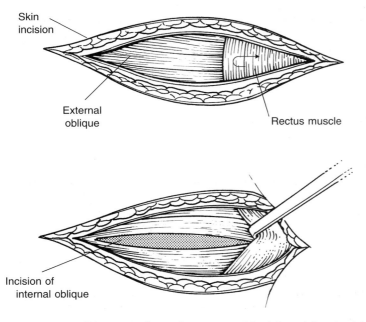

Fig. 13.7 Appendicectomy: lateral pararectal incision. After incision of the external oblique and anterior rectus sheath retract the rectus muscle medially and incise the internal oblique/posterior rectus sheath to expose the peritoneum.

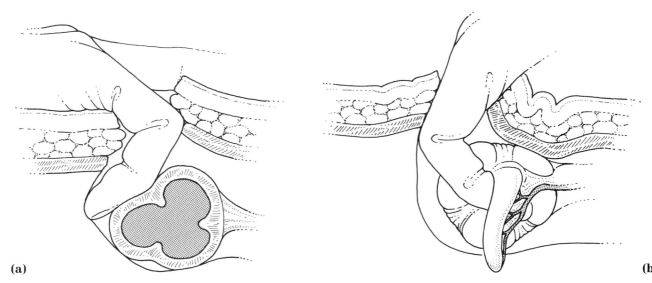

(a)   (b)

Fig. 13.8 To find the appendix insert a finger with the pulp laterally and slide it down the lateral aspect of the peritoneal cavity to find the caecum **(a)**. Rotate your finger and try to identify and hook up the appendix, which is at the lower pole of the caecum **(b)**.

> If you experience difficulty, or if the caecum is thickened and rigid, do not hesitate to extend the wound so that you can see the necessary structures and free them from inflammatory adhesions.

> If you pull out a loop of small bowel, replace it and try to push it medially with a swab in a sponge holder. Try again with your finger more laterally.

Centre your fascial incision over the linea semilunaris and incise the external oblique aponeurosis and anterior rectus sheath in the line of their fibres. Retract the lateral edge of the rectus muscle medially and incise the internal oblique aponeurosis and any posterior rectus sheath in the line of the previous incision (Fig. 13.7).

Diathermy any blood vessel that crosses this incision. This lateral pararectal incision is easier to make, less likely to bleed and easier to close than the standard muscle-splitting gridiron incision. It is rarely necessary to separate or divide internal oblique muscle fibres.

Insert a finger into the wound. Slide it laterally along the peritoneum and down the lateral abdominal wall and try to feel the caecum and/or appendix. If this latter is inflamed it will feel like a small sausage. If there are adhesions around the appendix, gently separate these with your finger and hook the appendix up into the incision (Fig. 13.8). When you have identified the appendix grasp it with a Babcock forceps to bring the appendix and the base of the caecum into the wound.

Elevate the appendix in one or two Babcock forceps and divide the mesoappendix. Push a clip through a translucent part of the mesoappendix, avoiding any blood vessels. Then apply the clip across the tissue, before dividing between the clip and the appendix. Repeat this once or twice to divide the whole mesoappendix.

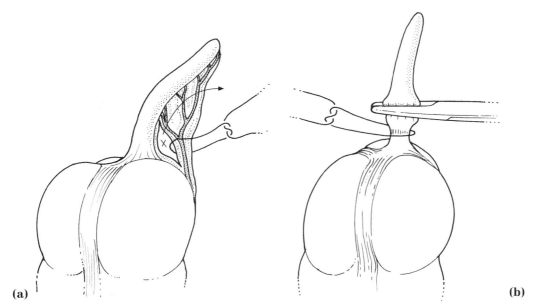

Fig. 13.9 **(a)** Divide the mesoappendix close to the serosa of the appendix base (X). Place one or more clips to secure the mesoappendix before dividing it between the clips and the appendix (arrow). Take care to enclose all the vessels in the clip to avoid troublesome bleeding. **(b)** Apply a small artery clip to the base of the appendix, release it and reapply it 5 mm distally. Ligate the base of the appendix in the groove of crushed tissue.

Apply a clip across the base of the appendix. Release the clip and move it 5 mm towards the tip and reapply. Tie a heavy ligature of catgut or Vicryl around the base of the appendix, in the groove made by the first application of your clip (Fig. 13.9). Cut the ligature with the ends long enough to grasp subsequently when you wish to invert the appendix stump. Cut across the appendix with a scalpel, between the tie and the clip, using the clip as a guide. Hand the appendix and instruments to the scrub nurse in a 'dirty' dish. Wipe the base of the appendix and the wound edges with a swab soaked in povidone iodine, then invert the stump of the appendix using a simple Z stitch (Fig. 13.10). This is quicker to use than a purse string, and avoids the need to pass the suture close to the vessels in the mesoappendix.

Check the base of the appendix and mesoappendix for haemostasis.

Allow the caecum to fall back into the wound, and pass a Poole sucker down the right side wall of the pelvis into the pouch of Douglas, to aspirate any exudate. This manoeuvre helps to prevent

> Make sure that you divide the appendicular artery close to the wall of the caecum, in order to avoid troublesome bleeding later (Fig. 13.9).

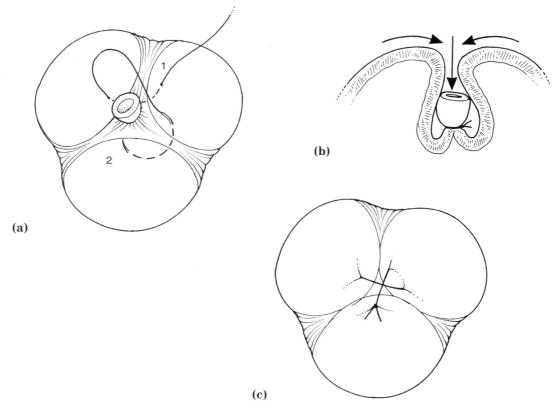

Fig. 13.10 **(a)** Pass a stitch through two convenient folds of serosa on one side of the appendix (1) and then on the opposite side (2). Grasp the ends of the ligature on the appendix stump in the tips of a small artery forceps and push it into the caecum. **(b)** Tie the stitch over the appendix stump and remove the artery forceps. **(c)** This shows the combined movements of inversion of the appendix stump and apposition of the serosa of the caecum by the suture.

> Do not rummage around the pelvis with swabs. This is an inefficient way of removing exudate and may cause abrasions leading to tubal fibrosis and infertility.

the formation of a pelvic abscess and you will be surprised on occasions how much purulent fluid is present.

Rapid bleeding from the pelvis

Blood in the pelvis is most likely to be due to a ruptured ovarian cyst. An ectopic pregnancy is less likely but a much more serious condition. Summon expert assistance immediately. Enlarge the incision medially, cutting rectus muscle if necessary, to give good access to the pelvic organs. If you can, control bleeding with large soft clamps and await the arrival an expert opinion before making a decision about ovarian or tubal preservation.

If you suspect or discover other more serious pathology summon senior assistance.

Wound closure

Close the wound with continuous absorbable suture such as Vicryl. Lift up the peritoneum/internal oblique/transversalis fascia with a clip on each side. Retract the rectus muscle medially and close the layer with a continuous stitch as far as the muscle belly. Release the rectus muscle and close the anterior sheath/external oblique fascia with a continuous suture.

Close the skin wound with a subcuticular suture and give the patient appropriate antibiotic prophylaxis according to your local protocol.

Aftercare

Allow the patient free fluids by mouth after recovery from the anaesthetic and encourage early mobilization. Most patients with acute appendicitis can be discharged home from hospital after 2–3 days.

> The commonest problem in appendicitis is failure to confirm the diagnosis. Deliver the small bowel through the wound for a distance of 75 cm to exclude a Meckel's diverticulum. Pass the sucker into the pelvis to aspirate fluid. If the pelvis is clear there is unlikely to be pelvic pathology and it is unnecessary to make prolonged attempts to deliver the right ovary into the wound. Pass the sucker up either side of the ascending colon to look for exudate, bile or intestinal contents, which could indicate cholecystitis or a perforated duodenal ulcer. If these examinations are negative, close the wound.

LAPAROTOMY INCISION AND CLOSURE

Make a laparotomy incision using the techniques described in Chapter 1. Site the incision and orientate it according to your consultant's preference. Incise skin with a knife and divide subcutaneous fat with the cutting diathermy. Use coagulation diathermy to cut muscle. Proceed with caution as you approach the peritoneum. Elevate the wound edges and make a small incision in the peritoneum. Air will enter and the bowel will fall away from the abdominal wall. Ensure that you have adequate length in the incision to examine the abdomen fully, to deal with the pathology you have found and to perform the procedures that were planned.

Before closure, check all the areas you have exposed, to make sure no swabs or instruments have been left behind and to confirm good haemostasis. Confirm that the swab, needle and instrument counts are correct. Close all abdominal incisions with a continuous full thickness closure with monofilament non-absorbable material (e.g. nylon or polypropylene). Select a large needle sufficient to take a comfortable 1 cm bite through all layers of the abdominal wall (except skin). Begin at the end of the incision furthest from your domi-

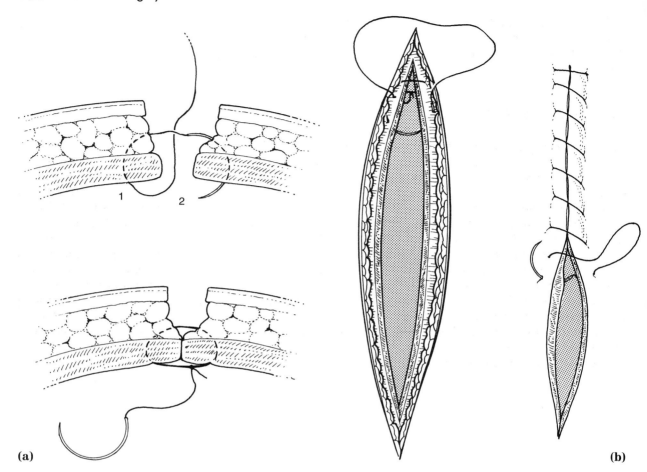

(a)   (b)

Fig. 13.11 Abdominal closure. **(a)** Start by passing the needle from within the abdominal cavity through the muscular layers (1). Complete the first suture by returning to the abdominal cavity (2) and tie a knot. **(b)** Pass once more from within to without and ask your assistant to hold the loop of thread away from you. Work towards yourself, taking full-thickness bites of each edge and pulling the loop through after each bite that comes to the outside. Avoid excessive tension.

nant hand. Pass the needle from within out and from without in and tie the knot on the inside. This avoids leaving a potentially troublesome knot in the subcutaneous tissue. Next bring the needle through all the layers of fascia and muscle to exit in the subcutaneous fat on the side of the wound away from your dominant hand. Pull the thread through and ask your assistant to hold it out of the way without tension. You are now ready to run along the full length of the wound taking bites of about 1 cm from the edge at 1 cm intervals (Fig. 13.11).

Each time the needle has passed in and out of the wound ensure that the loop is held away from the wound to avoid knotting the thread. Close the skin with a subcuticular suture as described in Chapter 1.

ACCESS FOR LAPAROSCOPY

All laparoscopic procedures require the creation of a pneumoperitoneum. The safest way to achieve this is by open incision. This is particularly true after previous surgery when adhesions may be present.

Place the anaesthetized patient supine on the operating table. It is not necessary to tilt the table. Ask for a medium-sized curved blade (No. 20). In a thin patient make a 1.5 cm vertical incision in the umbilicus, extending slightly below it. In an obese patient make a 1.5–2 cm slightly curved infraumbilical incision as close to the umbilicus as possible. Deepen the incision until you see the white fibres of the linea alba. Within the umbilicus the layers are very close and you will come to the fibrous tissue immediately.

Divide the fibres of the linea alba vertically in the midline under direct vision. Incise for 12–15 mm. This facilitates placement of the cannula and opening of the peritoneum. Apply a clip to each side of

> In an obese patient it may be difficult to confirm visually that you have entered the peritoneum. After you have elevated the fascia incise the next layer and then turn the knife round and drop the handle through the incision. If it descends easily you have entered the peritoneal cavity. Be careful not to let go of the knife handle! Take the knife out and insert a finger into the wound to confirm that it is within the peritoneal cavity.

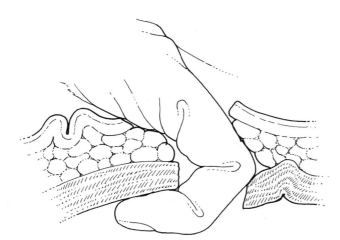

Fig. 13.12 To ensure that you have entered the abdominal cavity and to exclude adhesions to the anterior abdominal wall, pass a finger into the incision and rotate it while feeling the smooth slippery surface of the peritoneum. If you experience any resistance, proceed with extreme caution to avoid damaging bowel.

the incision in the fascia and ask your assistant to lift one while you lift the other away from the operating table. This creates a negative intra-abdominal pressure. Incise the peritoneum under direct vision and observe the abdominal contents falling away from the peritoneum. Extend the peritoneal excision to match the fascial incision and insert your finger to confirm that you have entered the peritoneum and that there are no adjacent adhesions; sweep it round through 360°. This should be easy to do, and you will feel the smooth peritoneal surface against your finger (Fig. 13.12). Any resistance suggests adhesions and you must proceed with caution.

Take a heavy monofilament suture (such as 0 polypropylene) on a J-shaped needle, pick up one edge of the fascial incision near its lower end and repeat on the opposite edge. Pass the needle on each occasion from within to without. Try to include the peritoneal layer if

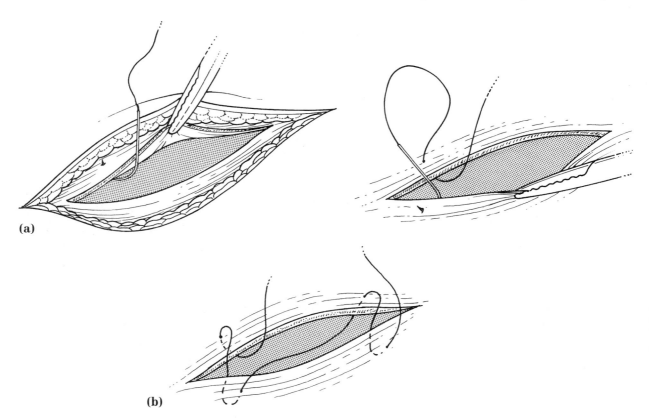

(a)

(b)

Fig. 13.13 Placement of a Z stitch at open access for a laparoscope. **(a)** Elevate one edge of the fascia with a clip and pass a J-needle through the fascial layer, retrieving the needle from the subcutaneous fat. Repeat this action on the opposite side of the wound. **(b)** Two further passes at the other end of the incision create a Z stitch, which will close the incision around the laparoscopic cannula.

possible and rotate the needle holder to bring the curve of the needle to the fat and into the wound (Fig. 13.13).

Pick it up with heavy forceps and withdraw it from the incision. Repeat this process near the upper end of the incision to create a Z stitch.

Take a 10mm cannula with a blunt obturator, or without an obturator, and insert it into the abdomen between the upper and lower limbs of your suture. It is helpful, but not essential, to use a Hassan cannula. This has a conical obturator that fits into the abdominal wound and helps seal it. An ordinary cannula can be used, by pulling the thread tight and crossing the ends once before bringing them around the cannula above the trumpet valve. Secure the ends with a clip and leave them long. This suture will serve to close the umbilical incision at the end of the procedure.

Verify that the cannula moves freely within the abdominal cavity then connect the gas supply and open the tap. Pass the laparoscope through the cannula and you are ready to inspect the abdominal contents and insert secondary ports.

INSERTION OF PORTS UNDER DIRECT VISION

Advance the laparoscope up to the abdominal wall to transilluminate it at a suitable point. Look for blood vessels. Take a solution of dilute bupivacaine and infiltrate the abdominal wall from the skin to the peritoneum at the proposed site. Withdraw the camera from the abdominal wall and press at the proposed site to confirm that it is suitable. You may see the needle and the local anaesthetic enter the peritoneal cavity. This is not significant. Simply withdraw the needle slightly and infiltrate beneath the peritoneum. Next, incise the skin making the incision slightly larger than the cannula diameter. Hold the cannula in your hand so that the end of the trocar rests against the adductor pollicis muscle. Press the whole assembly through the abdominal wall with a smooth, gradually increasing force, and observe the entry site within the abdomen using the laparoscope. Ensure that the tip of the trocar does not damage any underlying organ.

> Angle the line of the cannula during introduction to correspond with the optimum position of the cannula in use, i.e. pointing directly at the proposed site of operation. This will minimize difficulty with relocating instruments during the procedure.

LAPAROSCOPIC CLOSURE

After completion of a laparoscopic procedure withdraw all instruments under laparoscopic vision. Ensure that graspers and scissors are closed within your field of view and then follow them out through the cannula. Withdraw the cannula, observing the internal opening, to check for bleeding. Before finally withdrawing the laparoscope, deflate the pneumoperitoneum and check that all the internal openings are free of herniation. Slide the cannula up the laparoscope before you withdraw the scope. Then slowly come out of the abdominal wall, checking that there is no injured bowel attached to the cannula site, that no bowel herniates into the incision and that there is no bleeding. Close any incision for 10 mm or larger cannulas with a Z stitch like the one used for open access. Close the skin with Steri-Strips over 5 mm cannula sites and one or two interrupted subcuticular sutures for larger incisions.

VARICOSE VEINS

Many patients with varicose veins can be managed without operation. Patients with minimal varicosities, venous flares and whose main complaint is aching should be advised to use graduated elastic compression stockings. Patients with varicosities below the knee and without obvious saphenofemoral incompetence are best managed by sclerotherapy.

Injection sclerotherapy

Ask the patient to stand for a few minutes to make the varices prominent. Next ask him/her to step on to a 60 cm platform beside an examination couch. Ensure that you have some syringes already filled with 0.5 ml sodium tetradecyl sulphate and fitted with an orange injection needle. Place a strip of adhesive tape across the barrel of each syringe.

> Do not use more than four injections on each leg.

Warn the patient that any extravasation of injection may be painful and may cause permanent brown staining of the skin. Record the fact that you have given this warning in the notes.

With the patient still standing, insert a needle with syringe attached into a distal varix. Aspirate blood but do not inject at this time. Fix the syringe to the skin with the adhesive tape. Apply a second syringe in the same way although more proximally and work up towards the knee until you have reached a maximum of four syringes. Ask the patient to sit down on the couch, to lie flat and raise the leg you are treating. Ask an assistant to hold the heel to keep the leg at 30–45°. This empties blood from the veins and avoids dilution of the sclerosant. With a finger or thumb resting gently over the needle inject slowly from the most proximal syringe. If you feel the injection enter the subcutaneous tissues stop the injection at once. When the syringe is empty apply firm pressure with a piece of precut sponge and tape it to the leg. Remove the syringe and needle and repeat the process with the remaining syringes. When this has been done, and without lowering the foot, apply a compression bandage of elasticized crepe from the foot to the knee to ensure firm compression of all the injection sites. Cover this with an elastic stocking and ask the patient to lower the legs to the floor, stand up, and then to walk around for 10 min. This serves to dilute any sclerosant that has entered the deep veins, and reduces the risk of deep venous thrombosis. Repeat this process in the other leg if necessary.

Instruct the patient to keep the compression undisturbed for 48 hours, and to wear elastic stockings for a minimum of 10 days or according to your local hospital protocol.

Surgical treatment

Patients with extensive or large varicosities will require multiple avulsions. This is usually associated with saphenofemoral ligation and stripping of the long saphenous vein. Unless instructed otherwise by your consultant, strip the long saphenous vein from the groin down to the knee in patients with saphenofemoral incompetence.

Single leg varicose veins can be dealt with under local anaesthetic with a femoral nerve block. However, general anaesthetic is preferred by most patients and surgeons. Place the patient supine with the legs straight and the feet separated by at least 60 cm. This will require placement of a board across the lower end of the table. Separation of the feet opens up the groin and makes dissection there easier.

Have an assistant hold the foot of the leg(s) to be operated in the air while you prepare the skin from below the ankle to above the groin. It is easier for the assistant if you delay the head-down tilt until after the drapes have been placed. If this is a bilateral procedure, have a second assistant paint the other leg at the same time. Place a large sterile sheet beneath the leg (and over the other one if this is a one-leg procedure) and pull this sheet as far up under the leg as possible. Take a small sterile sheet folded so that it is about 10–15 cm across and 30 cm long. Tuck this between the legs to cover the genitalia. Place a towel across the abdomen to form the upper limit of the operative field. If necessary place towels laterally to provide lateral margins.

Incise in the groin following the skin crease and centring the incision 2.5 cm below and lateral to the pubic tubercle (Fig. 13.14).

Apply an Allis forceps to the dermis of each edge of the incision and ask your assistant to hold up one while you hold up the other. With scissors, incise the fatty tissue until you come on to the glistening blue saphenous vein. Deepen the incision equally along its length. You can

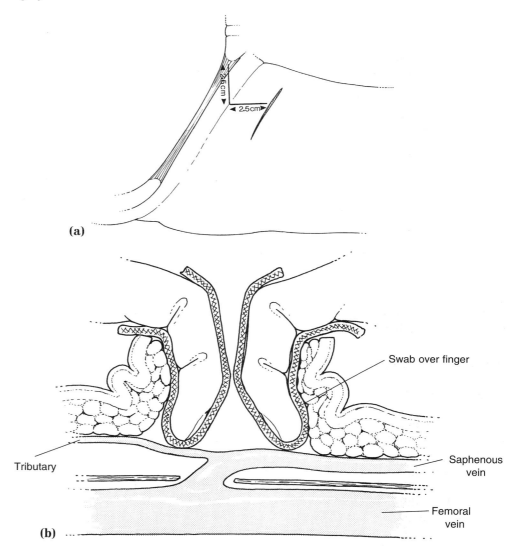

Fig. 13.14 (a) Centre the incision 2.5 cm lateral to and below the pubic tubercle. **(b)** When the saphenous vein is exposed, develop the plane in front of the vein and its tributaries by firm outward pressure with a finger covered by a small swab. This gives rapid bloodless separation in the correct plane.

now sweep the two wound edges away from the vein using a swab held over the index finger of each hand as shown in Fig. 13.14.

Clean the saphenous vein and identify all its tributaries up to the saphenofemoral junction. It is quicker to complete the dissection and then apply clips rather than to repeatedly clip and cut vessels in alternation with dissection. However, sometimes you will find it more

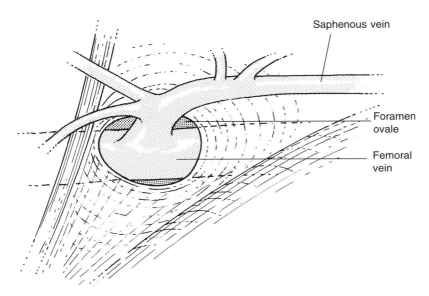

Saphenous vein

Foramen ovale

Femoral vein

Fig. 13.15   Identification of the saphenofemoral junction. It is essential to recognize the defect in the deep fascia, with the saphenous vein passing through it and joining the femoral vein beneath.

convenient to divide some of the tributaries to allow access to the saphenofemoral junction.

Sweep the fatty tissue off the saphenous vein to demonstrate the foramen ovale, which is the landmark of the saphenofemoral junction. Do not clip or divide any large vein until you have identified this landmark and confirmed that the saphenous vein enters the femoral vein beneath it (Fig. 13.15).

Apply two clips to all the tributaries of the saphenous vein and divide between the clips. Tie all these vessels with absorbable suture material. Clip the long saphenous vein securely and divide it 2–3 cm from the saphenofemoral junction. Gently pull the proximal stump laterally to expose any medial tributaries from the pudendal vessels entering the femoral vein. If you see these, carefully ligate them. Pass a right-angled Lahey forceps beneath the vessel and place a ligature in the jaws of the forceps. Withdraw the ligature around the vessel and tie it (Fig. 13.16).

When you have divided the saphenous vein hold it up vertically and place a strong tie around the saphenofemoral junction at the level of the foramen ovale.

> Do not cut the vein short, as a long stump will prevent the tie from rolling off the saphenous vein stump.

Stripping the long saphenous vein

Apply gentle traction on the saphenous vein using the clip you applied before dividing it. Make a small incision across part of the

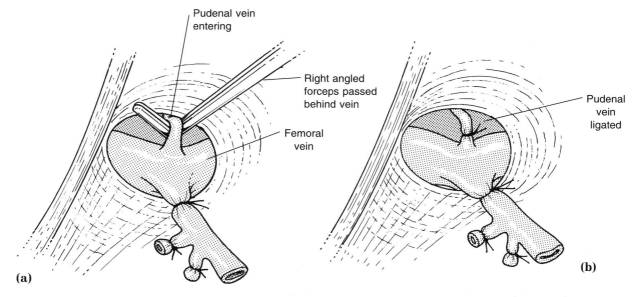

Fig. 13.16 Pull the saphenous vein stump laterally to expose the medial aspect of the femoral vein. Occasionally a pudendal vein enters here. If this is not ligated, recurrent varices may arise. Pass a right-angled clamp beneath the vein. Grasp a tie with this clamp and pull it round behind the vein, then tie the vein securely. It is not necessary to divide the pudendal vein; it may be dangerous to do so close to the femoral vein.

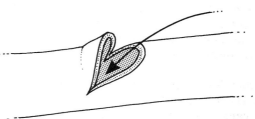

Fig. 13.17 Incision of a vein to allow cannulation. Make an angled cut part way across, to raise a distally based flap. It is then straightforward to feed the stripper wire down the vein.

circumference of the vein with scissors to raise a distally based flap (Fig. 13.17).

Pass the wire of the stripper down the long saphenous vein until you can feel it just below and behind the medial condyle of the tibia. Make a small skin incision over the vein and expose it by spreading the tips of a forceps in the subcutaneous tissue. Grasp the vein and the stripper, lift them up into the wound and cut down on to the stripper wire to expose it. Apply a clip to the distal part of the vein below the exit incision and divide the vein. Tie off the distal end.

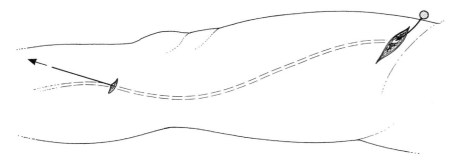

Fig. 13.18 View of the right leg with the stripper in place. Traction on the stripper in the axis of the leg will pull the vein down and out of the incision just below the medial aspect of the knee.

Pass a tie around the saphenous vein at its proximal end to hold the vein securely against the stripper wire. Attach a 1 cm olive to the proximal end of the wire and a handle to the distal end. Apply traction in the long axis of the leg to pull the stripper down through the thigh and out through the skin at the knee (Fig. 13.18).

Multiple avulsions

Minor varicosities related to the long saphenous may be sufficiently dealt with by stripping the vein, but most patients have distant varicosities or numerous vessels, which must be avulsed to avoid postoperative thrombophlebitis.

Preoperative marking   Ask the patient to stand for at least 1 min to fill the varices. Use an indelible black marker that will resist the skin preparation. Trace the course of every enlarged vein with a single line of the pen until all the veins that you wish to remove have been marked.

Operation   After you have completed saphenofemoral disconnection, proceed to avulsion. Use a small, straight, sharp-pointed blade (No. 11) and make single stab incisions beside the marks you have made, at intervals of 6–8 cm.

When you have made all the incisions, take a pair of small-toothed Kocher's forceps and insert the points into an incision. Spread them and advance them open to grasp the vein. Close the forceps on the vein and gently withdraw it from the wound (Fig. 13.19).

While pulling, use a gentle circular motion to tease out the vein from the incision. If more than 2 cm of vein emerges, grasp the vein with a mosquito or Dunhill forceps, apply one forceps to each limb of

> Make all the incisions before commencing avulsion, as your skin marks will be easier to see, and they may be washed off if there is much bleeding.

> Do not incise through the skin marks, as this risks tattooing the leg.

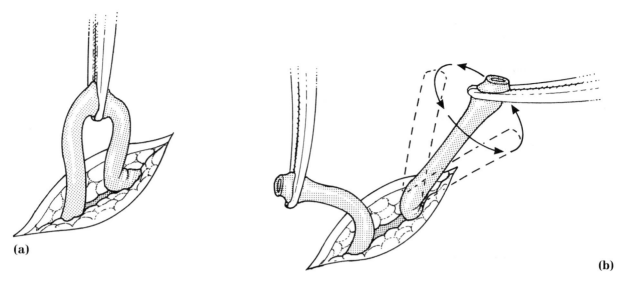

(a)

(b)

Fig. 13.19   Grasp the vein with the toothed Kocher's forceps and pull it through the small incision. Apply small artery forceps to each limb of the vein and cut between them. Then gently pull on each end in turn to extract as much length as possible. A circular rocking motion will help to free the vein.

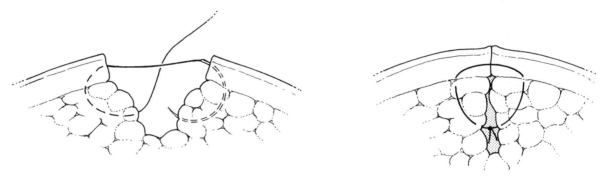

Fig. 13.20   Interrupted subcuticular stitch. Take a subcuticular bite on one side, starting on the deep aspect of the skin. Return to the deep aspect on the second side and tie the knot so that it lies in the subcutaneous tissue. Make sure the threads issue from the wound on the same side of the suture. If they cross the suture the stitch will be difficult to tie and will not close properly.

the vein and continue the process of avulsion. If the vein snaps, insert the Kocher's into the wound and try to retrieve as much vein as possible through each incision.

Skin closure   The wounds from avulsions require only Elastoplast dressings if they are sited in Langer's lines. If a wound gapes, appose the edges with Steri-Strips.

Close the longer incision at the knee where the vein was stripped with two subcutaneous Dexon or undyed Vicryl sutures, with the knot buried deeply (Fig. 13.20).

Close the groin incision with interrupted absorbable sutures in the subcutaneous fat and a subcuticular stitch in the skin. Apply Elastoplast dressings over all the incisions on the leg and then apply a firm crepe bandage from toe to upper thigh. This bandage can be removed the following day before the patient is discharged home from the ward. Give the patient a pair of elastic stockings to wear for 10 days to minimize swelling and bruising.

EXCISION OF BREAST LUMP

There are three types of breast lump that require surgical excision. The technique differs slightly according to the likely diagnosis.

Fibroadenoma

This lesion is well encapsulated, relatively mobile and can be excised without any surrounding normal tissue. Hold the lump firmly between a finger and thumb, to prevent it moving away from the incision. Incise over the lesion along its longest length, but orientate the incision to give the best cosmetic results. Above and below the nipple use a transverse incision, laterally use a radial incision (Fig. 13.21).

Incise through the breast tissue with the scalpel until you see the surface of the fibroadenoma. Take a small pair of scissors and dissect

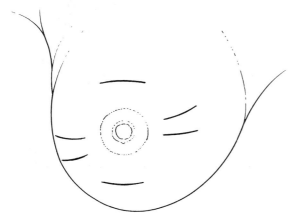

Fig. 13.21 Transverse orientation of the incision gives the best cosmetic results in the breast.

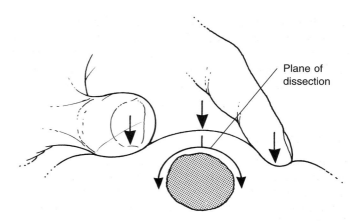

Plane of
dissection

Fig. 13.22   Excision of fibroadenoma. Apply downward pressure with finger and thumb on either side of the lesion and maintain this position to fix the lump until it is delivered into the wound. Cut down to the surface and then develop a plane around the lesion using scissors and blunt dissection.

around the surface of the lesion, alternately spreading the blades and dividing any fibrous attachments to the lesion. Maintain the fibroadenoma in position with a finger and thumb of your non-dominant hand throughout (Fig. 13.22).

As the fibroadenoma becomes freed from surrounding tissue, depress the skin on each side to deliver the lump into the wound. Complete the dissection on the deep surface. Apply diathermy to any bleeding points and close the wound with a subcuticular Dexon stitch.

Fibroadenosis

Excision of an area of benign fibroadenosis is rarely required if careful assessment with clinical examination, mammography and cytology all suggest benign disease. When doubt exists, excise the lesion for paraffin histology.

Make a radial, circumareolar or transverse incision as described above. Deepen the incision through the breast tissue until you reach the area of the lesion. Fibroadenosis is not mobile, and when you have deepened the incision to the nodular area you can grasp the hard breast tissue with a heavy forceps such as Bonney's. When you have done this, excise around the lesion with the knife to remove the area that has been worrying the patient. Do not attempt an extensive dissection, but try to remove the hard area that has caused concern. The wall of the cavity is likely to be white and fibrous, but there will be some bleeding points, which should be diathermied.

Do not put deep sutures into breast tissue. A better cosmetic result is achieved by skin closure alone. Ensure complete haemostasis with diathermy. Close the skin with a subcuticular Dexon suture. Apply a gauze dressing and ensure that the patient wears a firm and comfortable brassiere immediately after the operation. Drains are rarely necessary.

Malignant breast lump

Most cases of breast cancer can now be managed by excision of the primary lesion with subsequent radiotherapy to the breast and either surgery or radiotherapy to the axillary lymph nodes. Axillary dissection and techniques for removing screen-detected cancers are beyond the scope of this book.

If preliminary clinical assessment, mammography and cytology suggest that a lump is malignant, aim to remove it with 1 cm of surrounding normal tissue. Lumpectomy is appropriate if this will remove not more than one quadrant of the breast. Larger lesions require mastectomy. There is no definite upper size limit, because the decision for lumpectomy or mastectomy is influenced by the ratio between the size of the lesion and the size of the patient's breast.

Make an adequate incision, 1 cm longer than the lesion in each direction. Hold the lesion firmly between the finger and thumb of your non-dominant hand and incise through the breast tissue, aiming to take 1 cm of normal tissue in all directions around the lesion. Deepen the incision around the lesion on all sides until you can lift up a core of breast tissue with the contained lesion. When you can feel

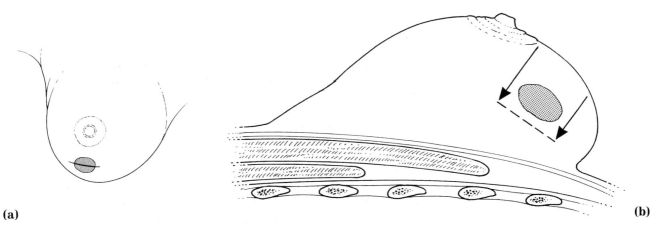

(a)   (b)

Fig. 13.23 Excision of a malignant breast lump. The incision should be longer than the lesion to allow an adequate margin of excision. Aim to excise a core of breast tissue around the lesion. Cut horizontally through the breast beneath the lump when you can feel the deep aspect between finger and thumb.

the deep surface, cut across the breast tissue beneath the lesion (Fig. 13.23).

It may be necessary to go down to the deep fascia for a deep lesion. Avoid unnecessary extension along the easy plane beneath the breast. This may lead to a conical cavity and increases scarring and deformity.

Ensure complete haemostasis by careful use of diathermy. It may be necessary to retract the wound edges with Langenbeck's forceps and pack the cavity with a swab. Gently displace the swab to demonstrate each bleeding point in turn. Ensure that all swabs are removed at the end of the operation.

Follow the usual practice of your consultant when deciding whether to suture or drain the cavity. Close the skin with a subcuticular suture as appropriate.

ABDOMINAL WALL HERNIA

There are four main types of hernia. Incisional hernia will not be considered here as its repair requires advanced surgical skills. Midline and femoral hernias are relatively straightforward to repair, whereas inguinal hernia is likely to recur unless you pay meticulous attention to detail and use a proven technique.

Midline hernia

These are commonly in the epigastrium or at the umbilicus. They should be repaired to prevent strangulation of the contained extraperitoneal fat or omentum. Small midline hernias are easily repaired under local anaesthetic. A large hernia may require a general anaesthetic.

Make a transverse incision slightly longer than the fat contained in the hernia. Deepen the incision with the scalpel through the subcutaneous tissue until you see the shining, orangey-yellow capsule of the hernia. Lift up the skin on each side with a skin hook and follow the plane around the hernia with forceps and scissors. In this situation it is permissible to insert the scissors and open them to dissect the plane. Mobilize the hernia completely and follow it down to the fascial defect. In epigastric hernias the defect is usually much smaller than the hernia itself.

Divide the attachments of the hernial sac to the defect in the fascia. Reduce the fat through the fascia, or apply an artery forceps and excise the surplus fat. Ligate the pedicle before releasing the artery forceps. When you can see the fascial ring with the hernial contents reduced or excised, incise the fascia laterally for 1 cm on each side

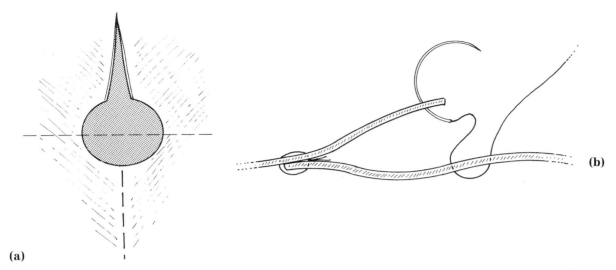

(a)

(b)

Fig. 13.24   Repair of midline hernia. **(a)** Incise the fascia perpendicular to the midline on both sides for 1 cm beyond the defect. **(b)** Place the first row of sutures so the knots are buried and the two edges overlap (see text). The overlapping repair is completed by interrupted sutures placed as shown.

(Fig. 13.24). This will enable you to overlap the two edges of the fascia in the horizontal plane.

Use a non-absorbable suture. For a small hernia two or three interrupted stitches will be sufficient. Pass the needle through the lower edge of the fascial defect near its free margin and then bring the needle through the upper edge at least 1 cm from its free border. Pass the needle back through the upper edge of the fascia and pick up the lower edge near its margin (Fig. 13.24). Place all of this first row of sutures before tying them. When you tie the sutures, the knots will be beneath the upper edge of the fascia, and the free edge will overlap the lower leaf. Next suture the free edge of the upper leaf to the superficial aspect of the lower leaf of the fascia (Fig. 13.24).

Subcutaneous sutures are not necessary. Suture the skin with a subcuticular stitch.

Femoral hernia

Femoral hernia may present as an emergency with strangulation, or electively as a variable swelling in the groin, below the inguinal ligament. Femoral hernia should be repaired at an early date because of the high risk of strangulation.

You can use a low approach, in the groin below the inguinal ligament. For this, local anaesthesia is satisfactory. You will not be

> When dealing with an umbilical hernia, make the incision slightly curved, around the lower margin of the umbilicus. Dissect the skin off the deep tissue and repair the hernia.

> When you have sutured the skin of an umbilical hernia, fold up a dressing swab four or five times to create a small pack. Tuck this into the umbilicus and apply a standard absorbent adhesive dressing over the top. This will compress the skin of the umbilicus against the deep tissue and recreate a normal appearance.

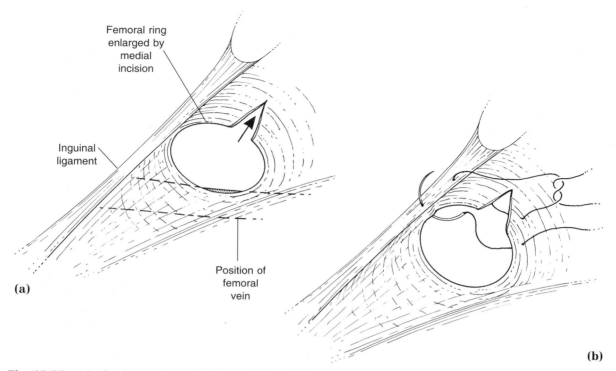

Fig. 13.25 **(a)** The femoral canal after excision of the sac. Note the medial extension to allow reduction of the contents. **(b)** Place a series of interrupted sutures to approximate the anterior and posterior aspects of the femoral canal.

Enlarge the neck of the sac by incising the femoral ring. Remember the vein is lateral, and incise the femoral ring medially. Diathermy any bleeding from the pudendal artery. Enlarge the ring sufficiently to reduce the contents of the sac, then excise the sac at the level of the femoral ring.

able to resect gangrenous bowel or deal with an associated inguinal hernia through this approach.

Infiltrate the groin with dilute lignocaine. Verify the position of the inguinal ligament and make an incision 1 cm below this and parallel to it. Begin over the femoral artery, avoiding the femoral nerve more laterally. Deepen the incision over the hernia, and develop the plane between the hernial sac and surrounding tissue. Identify the inguinal ligament above the sac. Mobilize the sac toward its neck and inject more local anaesthetic into the neck of the sac and the femoral canal (Fig. 13.25).

Incise the sac to inspect its contents. Apply two clips to the sac and cautiously divide between them. When you have entered the sac, mop up any fluid with a swab and extend the incision. Omentum may be excised (with ligation of its pedicle) but any bowel in the hernia should be reduced. Necrotic bowel that requires resection must be dealt with through an abdominal incision.

Repair the hernia using two (or occasionally three) interrupted sutures of 0 nylon. Pass the needle through the femoral ring posteriorly and bring it out anteriorly through the femoral ring/inguinal ligament. Do not tie any sutures until all have been placed.

Subcutaneous sutures are not required. Close the skin with a subcuticular monofilament. Aim to mobilize the patient as soon as possible. After emergency repair, or for a large hernia, give one dose of intravenous antibiotics and leave a suction drain in the wound for 24 hours.

Inguinal hernia

Inguinal hernia is common in men of all ages. A hernia can usually be repaired under local anaesthetic unless it is very large. Inguinoscrotal hernias that can be fully reduced are suitable for repair under local anaesthetic. There are two widely used techniques for repair of inguinal hernia: the mesh (Lichtenstein) repair and the Shouldice repair. You should not attempt to perform these operations without supervision until you have considerable experience.

Mesh repair

Infiltrate the skin with lignocaine 0.5%. Use 10 ml to cover the area of incision and subcutaneous tissue, and infiltrate 2 ml deep to the external oblique to block the ilioinguinal nerve (Chapter 2). Infiltrate a further 2 ml around the pubic tubercle.

Make a skin incision 5–7 cm in length, above the inguinal ligament, slightly curved and lying in a skin crease. The medial end of the incision should be 2–3 cm above the pubic tubercle.

Deepen the incision with a knife through subcutaneous fat and Scarpa's fascia. Do not be fooled into thinking you have reached the external oblique when you have got only as far as Scarpa's fascia. On the way, you will divide the superficial inferior epigastric vein. This may require clips and a ligature but can usually be controlled with diathermy. When you have reached the fascia you will recognize its white, glistening fibres. Expose the fascia in the full length of the wound by lifting up the skin and subcutaneous tissue and cleaning off the fat from the fascia first with the knife blade and subsequently with a swab wrapped over your finger (Fig. 13.26).

Identify the superficial inguinal ring and incise the external oblique 5 cm from the ring, in the line of the fibres, so that extension along the line of the fibres will enter the superficial ring (Fig. 13.26). Pick up each edge of the external oblique with an artery clip, lift up the fascia and split its fibres with a partly opened pair of scissors. Insert the blades of the scissors into the defect in the fascia and, without

Remember that the femoral vein is lateral to the femoral canal. Put your non-dominant index finger on the vein while you place the stitches. Aim to close the canal snugly without compressing the vein.

If there is a high likelihood of strangulated bowel in the hernia, operate under general anaesthesia and use a high approach. This can be either lateral to the rectus (McEvedy) or transinguinal (Shouldice). The Shouldice repair (p. 302) allows good access to the femoral region and adequate exposure for bowel resection in most cases, and enables a more rapid recovery than the McEvedy approach.

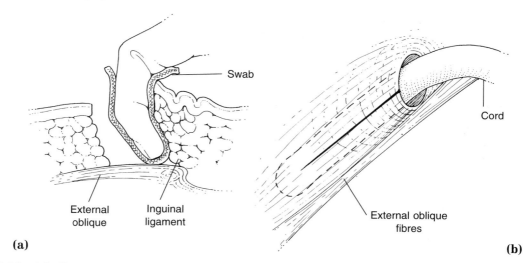

Fig. 13.26 **(a)** Clean the fat off the external oblique with a finger and swab. Make sure that you have exposed the glistening white fibres of the fascia to allow the correct plane to develop. **(b)** Incise the external oblique as shown to expose the length of the inguinal canal.

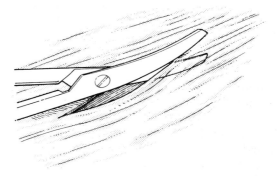

Fig. 13.27 When the fascia is exposed make a small excision in it and extend this by pushing the slightly opened blade of scissors along the line of the fibres. The scissors are held in a fixed position with the tips only slightly opened (inset).

closing the scissors, push along the line of the fibres in the direction you wish to go (Fig. 13.27).

Lift up the fascia on each side and separate it from the underlying internal oblique, transversalis and hernia. You may see the ilioinguinal nerve traversing the external oblique. If possible, preserve and protect it. If this is not possible, divide it cleanly beneath

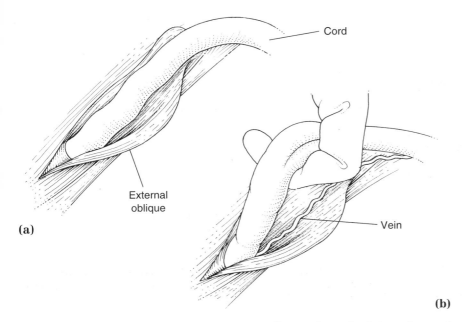

Cord

External
oblique

(a)

Vein

(b)

Fig. 13.28 **(a)** Dissect the cord by passing a finger along the internal aspect of external oblique towards the pubic tubercle, and lift the cord forward. **(b)** Hook the cord up with your finger and divide any cremasteric vein that runs behind the cord on the fascia.

the external oblique. It is wise to inject 1 ml lignocaine into the nerve proximal to the point of division before you divide it.

Lift up the lower leaf of external oblique and insert your finger between the fascia and the cord. Slide your finger downward, medially and backwards to run behind the cord and up towards the pubic tubercle (Fig. 13.28). Lift the cord up on your finger and make sure that you have lifted up all the cord tissue.

Lift the cord up over the index finger of your non-dominant hand. Make a small incision in the cremasteric fascia of the cord and extend this toward the deep ring. Straighten your finger, which lifts up the cord, and gently spread the cord tissues across your finger (Fig. 13.29).

Hold a swab in your dominant hand and gently push the cord tissues laterally across your non-dominant index finger. You are looking for the edge of a hernial sac in the cord (indirect hernia). This is usually quite obvious as a double fold of pearly white tissue (Fig. 13.29). When you see it, apply an artery clip to the very edge and lift it up. Inject more local anaesthetic into the cord at the deep ring before you dissect the sac. Ask your assistant to hold the clip under

> When you dissect the cord away from the posterior wall, ensure that all the fascial attachments are divided down to the deep ring so that the cord is fully mobile.

> You will usually see some cremasteric veins running close to the pubic tubercle on the posterior wall of the inguinal canal. Put a clip across the vein near the pubic tubercle and another one near the deep ring. Divide the vein between the clips and tie each end. This manoeuvre will add extra length to the cord and make sure you have a clean posterior wall (Fig. 13.28).

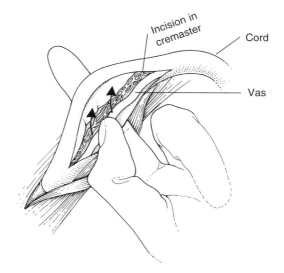

Fig. 13.29 After making an incision longitudinally in the cremaster, hold the cord over your index finger and with a swab held in the other hand spread out the cord tissues by lateral pressure (arrows). The edge of the sac will be evident as a longitudinal or crescentic fold of white tissue. Check that it is not a vein by releasing tension. The veins will fill with blood but the sac remains white.

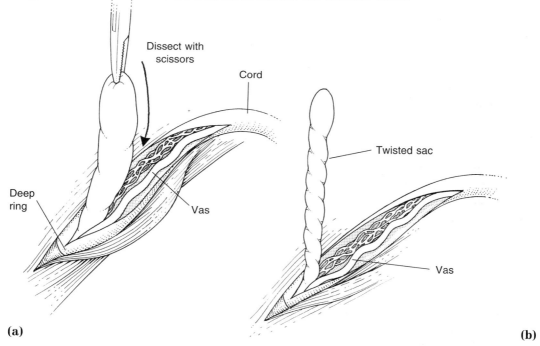

(a)

(b)

Fig. 13.30 **(a)** Lift the sac away from the vas and vein in the cord. Separate it with sharp dissection using scissors, until the sac is isolated down to the deep ring. **(b)** Before suture ligation of the sac, twist it to empty it of its contents.

gentle tension. Dissect the sac free with scissors, taking care not to injure any veins or the vas (Fig. 13.30).

Clean the sac down to the deep ring, where you will ligate it. First make sure that the sac is empty, either by opening it and passing a finger down to the deep ring, or by twisting it to force any contents back into the abdomen (Fig. 13.30). Pass a suture twice through the base of the sac close to the deep ring, as described in Chapter 1, and tie the suture securely. Cut across the sac and check its cut surface. Look for the glistening peritoneal surface and make sure there is no velvety pink mucosa present. If you see mucosa, call for senior assistance. If the sac appears clean it is safe to cut the suture. When you do this the neck of the sac should disappear inside the deep ring.

If there is a direct hernia this can be pressed down with a finger or a swab to demarcate the posterior wall. You are going to strengthen the posterior wall by applying a polypropylene mesh, sutured to the strong ligamentous margins of the inguinal canal.

> When you have mobilized the cord, inject some lignocaine into the deep ring before beginning dissection in the cord.

> When you have dissected the sac, inject some more local anaesthetic into the base of the sac before twisting, pulling or suturing it.

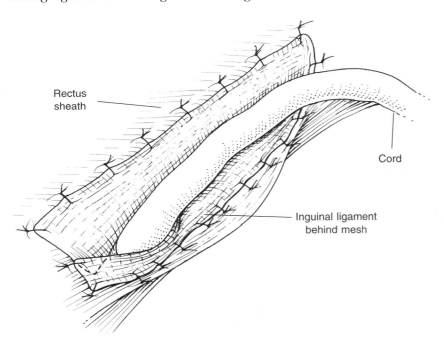

Fig. 13.31 Mesh repair. The mesh is placed behind the spermatic cord and sutured with a continuous stitch to the inguinal ligament, from the pubic tubercle to well lateral of the deep ring. The mesh overlies the lower part of the rectus sheath and the posterior wall of the inguinal canal and is wrapped laterally around the deep ring. Secure the upper edge with a few interrupted sutures.

In the presence of a large sac, divide the sac in the upper inguinal canal, taking care to stop all bleeding points on the distal cut edge. Do not attempt to remove a long inguinoscrotal sac if its contents can be reduced. Additional dissection causes extensive postoperative swelling in the scrotum.

If you have to dissect a sac distally in order to mobilize its contents, insert a suction drain into the scrotum and bring it out above the inguinal wound. This will help to reduce postoperative swelling.

If you are in the right plane, the yellow extraperitoneal fat will bulge into the incision. Apply a large curved artery clip (e.g. Sawtell) to the fat and allow the weight of the clip to push the fat back into the wound (Fig. 13.32).

Take an appropriate-sized piece of mesh, usually 12×8 cm, and tailor it to fit the inguinal canal. You may need to trim one corner where the mesh will lie over the inguinal ligament and pubic tubercle. Estimate the position of the deep ring and cut down to this level from one short edge of the mesh (Fig. 13.31).

Some surgeons use the added refinement of cutting a small disc to accommodate the cord at the site of the deep ring. This is not necessary unless the cord is very bulky.

With a 2/0 polypropylene stitch, attach one corner of the mesh to the fascia just above the pubic tubercle. Do not pass the stitch through the pubic tubercle as this causes postoperative pain. Continue the suture along the inguinal ligament, fixing the lower long edge of the mesh to the ligament (Fig. 13.31). Continue this suture well beyond the deep ring. Attach the medial and upper borders of the mesh with interrupted sutures to the rectus sheath and transversalis fascia. Laterally, overlap the two 'tails' of the mesh and suture them down snugly around the cord (Fig. 13.31).

Double-check that the patient has a single intravenous dose of broad-spectrum antibiotic before closing the external oblique aponeurosis with a continuous suture.

The skin wound should fall together comfortably without sutures. Insert a subcuticular stitch to close the skin.

Shouldice repair

The Shouldice repair is suitable for local or general anaesthesia. It is a well-tried and trusted technique that can be used for all types of inguinal hernia, including large direct and inguinoscrotal hernias. It is also an anatomically satisfying approach to a femoral hernia. The Shouldice repair of inguinal hernia allows pre-emptive closure of the femoral canal when an incipient femoral hernia is detected.

Proceed as described above for injection of local anaesthesia, mobilization of the cord and removal of an indirect sac.

Place an Allis forceps around the cord and pull it laterally. Incise the posterior wall of the inguinal canal in the same line as the external oblique incision. Begin this incision 1 cm medial to the deep ring to avoid the inferior epigastric vessels. The posterior wall often has two distinct layers: ensure you have cut through both and pick up both layers with a clip on each side of the incision. Extend the incision medially to just above the pubic tubercle. It is a mistake not to incise medially when the posterior wall appears sound. Failure to complete the incision leads to a medial weakness of the repair. As you extend medially you may need to apply a second pair of artery clips on the superior and inferior leaves of the transversalis fascia.

Hold up the two artery clips on the superior leaf of transversalis

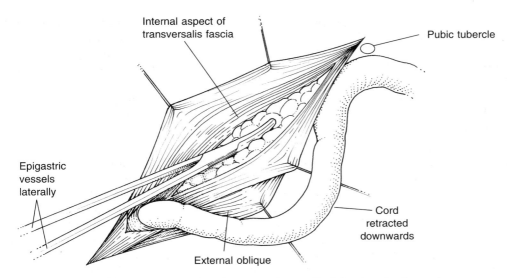

Internal aspect of
transversalis fascia

Pubic tubercle

Epigastric
vessels
laterally

Cord
retracted
downwards

External oblique

Fig. 13.32 Shouldice repair. Incise the posterior wall of the inguinal canal from the deep ring to the pubic tubercle. Take care not to injure the epigastric vessels laterally. Sweep the extraperitoneal fat down into the abdomen and hold it there with a heavy artery forceps. Hold up the upper leaf to expose the shining conjoint tendon and clean it along its length.

fascia. Sweep the extraperitoneal fat down off the fascia to expose its glistening white inner surface. Repeat this with the lower leaf. As you sweep the fat down towards the pelvis identify the femoral ring just lateral to and below the pubic tubercle and below the inguinal ligament. If the femoral ring is wide (1 cm or more) close it with two or three interrupted nylon sutures.

Extend the incision laterally in front of the epigastric vessels. Take care to sweep the vessels down away from the fascia before you divide it. Extend laterally into the deep ring and free the fascia around the cord.

You are now ready to begin the overlapping repair of the posterior wall. Use a monofilament nylon suture and go through the lower leaf of transversalis at the level of the pubic tubercle. Do not go through the pubic tubercle as this causes postoperative pain. Bring the suture out through the upper leaf of the fascia and tie it securely. Leave the end long (hold it down with a clip). Take another bite of the lower leaf and then pick up the inner aspect of the conjoint tendon. Hold the clip on the upper leaf vertically up from the patient to expose the glistening white fibres of the tendon and catch this with the needle, bringing it out on the inner aspect of the transversalis fascia. Repeat the process of picking up the free edge of the lower leaf and the inner aspect of the conjoint tendon (Fig. 13.33).

> This part of the operation is much easier if you divide all the attachments of the cord to the deep ring with scissors.

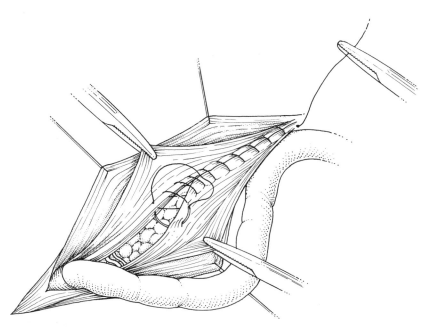

Fig. 13.33   Begin at the pubic tubercle and attach the lower leaf of the posterior wall to the inside of the conjoint tendon with a continuous polypropylene suture. Continue up to the deep ring.

Keep the extraperitoneal fat pushed down toward the pelvis by applying a large curved clip and using the weight of the clip to hold the fat down.

Continue this suture line towards the deep ring. Once you have got halfway, you can remove the clip holding down the extraperitoneal fat. Continue the closure up to the deep ring, until it fits snugly around the cord. Keep pulling the cord laterally until the posterior wall is closed. Tie a slip knot in the suture by pulling it through the last loop of the suture and snugging that down, repeated three times (Fig. 13.34).

Bring the needle out through the upper leaf of the transversalis fascia and catch the cut end of cremaster muscle in the cord. Suture these two bites down to firm tissue below the deep ring. This will be either the inguinal ligament or preferably the iliopubic tract which is a condensation of fascia lying parallel to but behind the inguinal ligament. Continue the suture back to the pubic tubercle, fixing the superior leaf to the iliopubic tract or inguinal ligament (Fig. 13.35). When the posterior wall has been completely double-breasted, tie the suture to the end previously left long at the pubic tubercle.

In the original description of this repair, a further two layers of sutures were inserted to reinforce the posterior wall, between conjoint tendon and the inguinal ligament. The external oblique layer

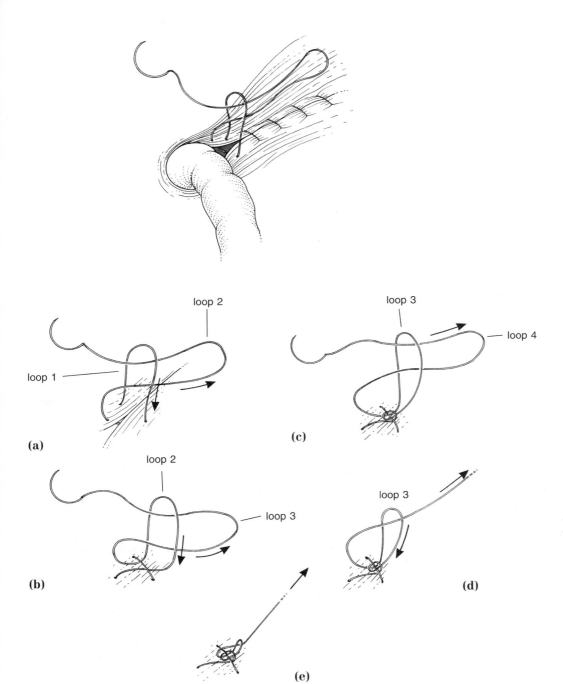

Fig. 13.34 Prevent the suture from loosening by tying a slip knot at the deep ring. Leave the last stitch loose (loop 1) and pull a loop of thread (2) through loop 1. Tension on loop 2 will pull down loop 1 over it. Pass another loop (3) through loop 2 and snug down loop 2 in the same way. This can be repeated (loops 3 and 4). Alternatively pass the needle through loop 3 and pull it down to complete the knot.

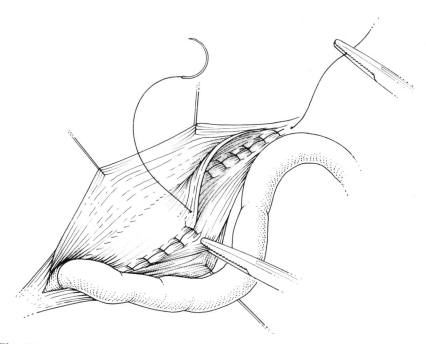

Fig. 13.35 After securing the stitch at the deep ring snugly around the cord, fold the upper leaf over your first suture line and attach it to the inguinal ligament, or the iliopubic tract just behind it, with a continuous suture. Carry this right down to the pubic tubercle and tie your stitch to the loose end from the beginning of your suture line.

was then double-breasted to provide added security. These additional layers are unnecessary. It is sufficient now to release the cord from the tissue forceps and close the external oblique over the cord. Before closing the fascia, fix the cremaster of the cord to the internal oblique or rectus sheath with one or two non-absorbable sutures. This helps to prevent the low-lying testis that can result from complete disconnection of the cremaster muscle. Close external oblique with a non-absorbable suture. Pick up the upper and lower edge of the fascia at the lateral extremity of the incision. Cut the loose end short and make a simple continuous suture as far medially as possible. Try to close the superficial ring snugly around the cord and carry the closure as far as the pubic tubercle to provide some support for the posterior wall repair in this region.

A subcutaneous suture is not necessary. Close the skin with a monofilament subcuticular suture.

Use generous volumes of dilute local anaesthetic to obtain adequate analgesia throughout the procedure.

At the end of the procedure, encourage the patient to mobilize and to believe in the strength of the repair by asking him to sit up on the operating table, step down on to the floor and walk out of the operating room to a waiting chair, which will take him back to the ward.

Index

Page numbers appearing in bold refer to figures and page numbers appearing in italics refer to tables